INSTANT CALM
IN THE AGE OF ANXIETY

When tension ties you in knots, you want help fast. This book, by a world-famous authority on stress-free living, offers the easiest, most effective relaxation techniques ever assembled in a single volume. They include age-old methods from many different cultures, and exercises from the most up-to-date scientific research. With the guidance of this book, you will be able to control your own stress level. Paul Wilson tells you how to make yourself calm and stress-free with simple exercises such as:

- Holding your hands in a relaxed position
- Massaging certain points on your head, leg, or arm
- Drinking hot water instead of tea or coffee

By removing your immediate anxiety, these techniques can help you regain perspective on life as a whole, enabling you to lower your tension level for the long term. If you want to feel better, sleep better, think better, and relate to others better from this moment on, this book is for you.

PAUL WILSON, author of the internationally acclaimed *The Calm Technique*, is one of the world's leading authorities on relaxation. He has written *Instant Calm* to answer the need of people who require swift relief from the pressure of stress before they can make relaxation a permanent part of their life. Chairman of a successful Sydney, Australia, advertising agency, he also works as a communications consultant and serves as director of a hospital. Wilson is a noted public speaker and the author of two novels.

INSTANT
CALM

*Over 100 Easy-to-Use Techniques for
Relaxing Mind and Body*

PAUL WILSON

A PLUME BOOK

PLUME
Published by the Penguin Group
Penguin Books USA Inc., 375 Hudson Street,
New York, New York 10014, USA
Penguin Books Ltd, 27 Wrights Lane,
London W8 5TZ, England
Penguin Books Australia Ltd, Ringwood,
Victoria, Australia
Penguin Books Canada Ltd, 10 Alcorn Avenue,
Toronto, Ontario, Canada M4V 3B2
Penguin Books (N.Z.) Ltd, 182–190 Wairau Road,
Auckland 10, New Zealand

Penguin Books Ltd, Registered Offices:
Harmondsworth, Middlesex, England

Published by Plume, an imprint of Dutton Signet,
a division of Penguin Books USA Inc.
First published in Australia by Penguin Books Australia Ltd

First Plume Printing, May, 1995

20

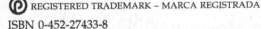

CONTENTS

PART THREE

LONGER-TERM CALM SOLUTIONS

PART FOUR

CRISIS

For Ron Wilson and Peter O'Brien

This book is dedicated to two men who, in a matter
of a few difficult months, taught me more about the
nature of healing and dealing with life's ills than years of
personal study and research.

Their beliefs and attitudes could not have been further
opposed: one probed the limits of alternative healing
while the other placed his trust in the conventional. Yet
both were inspirations, not only to me, but to all who
came in contact with them.

I have tried to assimilate some of the lessons of their
lives into this book.

*Have no fear,
you're going to feel much better
after reading this book.*

In this easily understood guide to calm and contentedness,
you will find more than a hundred fast-acting techniques that can be
of extraordinary comfort to you in your work, your home
and your relationships.

Some of these techniques have the capacity to revolutionise the way
you feel about worry, anxiety and nervousness. Others have the
capacity to neutralise the problems life throws at you.

Individually, they will give you strength to cope with the most
trying situations. Combined, they form an armoury of counterforces
to a competitive, insensitive and maybe even frightening world.

These are just some of the ways *Instant Calm* will work for you.

IN SEARCH OF CALM

It seems like half a lifetime ago I wrote a book called *the Calm Technique*.

It was intended as a no-nonsense, non-mystical guide to meditation: a way for ordinary people to learn how to relax; a simple, foolproof way of helping to cope with the stresses and anxieties of modern life.

It has grown into something much more.

While I'd always been confident there was a sizeable audience for such a work, the demand for *the Calm Technique* surpassed my most optimistic expectations – not only in this country, but all around the English-speaking world.

Sales have been great; the book has been adopted by so many authorities in the field – teachers of meditation, stress-management counsellors, medical practitioners, even a couple of talk-back radio heroes – that I often run into people who have just returned from such-and-such a health farm with a copy under their arm, or who have had it recommended by their doctor or psychiatrist.

I suppose I should be grateful. Yet, I still felt something about this process had not turned out the way I intended.

Accompanying any successful self-help book is the ubiquitous Speaker's Tour. In my case this involved not only a staggering number of evening addresses to stressed-out executives, but more 'alternative' venues than most people suspect even exist. I don't suppose there are many authors who have shared a stage with Indian mystics and a representative of the Dalai Lama on one night, and with high-powered representatives of our Top Ten Corporations the next. I did just that.

After several such occasions, it became apparent that those who needed the Calm Technique most were not the over-stressed business executives (who had no time for anything more complicated than a quick fix), nor the seekers of higher consciousness (who sought more spiritual or mystical depth than I was prepared to offer). The irony was that those who needed its techniques most were those who were least likely to use them.

Why?

Sometimes they lacked the patience to read an entire book. Other times they did not believe a programme of *any* sort could change their lives. Mostly, however, it was because their busy, stress-filled lifestyles could not accommodate the simple discipline of putting aside a half-hour or so each day to meditate.

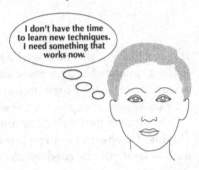

'Half an hour?' spluttered a highly stressed partner in a law firm. 'I can prepare half a case in half an hour.'

On another occasion, a young secretary from the business district in which I work was almost in tears as she explained: 'I don't have the time to learn new techniques; I need something that works now.'

These were not isolated incidents.

It seems that with the passing of each year our perseverance diminishes. Perhaps it is a by-product of the television age, the over-promotion of spectacular successes, or the result of our lives becoming more and more rushed and cramped. Perhaps it is the never-ending barrage of advertising and its 'If you want it, here it is, come and get it' mentality. Whatever the reason, one fact is clear: impatience is not only rife, but actually works *against* the effects we strive for when using the Calm Technique.

It is now obvious to me that the solution sought by so many worried, stressed and distressed people – everyday people suffering from everyday anxieties and problems – does not need to be as refined and as life-changing as the Calm Technique. What they need is something easier and more immediate.

Hence, *Instant Calm*.

A word about holism

Over the years I have researched and assembled a mind-boggling array of calming techniques for a book such as this. Yet, I hesitated before writing it.

The philosophy of a guide to instant relaxation – a compendium of quick fixes – seemed counter to what the Calm Technique had strived so earnestly to achieve. The Calm Technique is, after all, a holistic way of treating stress and tension, and such an approach insists that painful symptoms are simply your body's way of informing you of an ailment or condition; to treat the symptom is to ignore the condition that prompted it.

QUICK LIKE AN ASPIRIN

Unashamedly, this is a book of quick-fix solutions. Removal of the symptoms. Fast relief, with minimal regard for long-term cures.

'Just like aspirin,' I was reminded by an academic friend. 'It has no long-term curative role, either. Yet many people consider it one of this century's most important developments in healing.'

Aspirin. A quick solution. Effective, short-term relief from painful symptoms. Aspirin became my inspiration for *Instant Calm*.

Didn't holistic standards demand that stress and anxiety be treated in a similar way?

Herein lay the paradox. For the most part, holism depends on the body's ability to heal itself. Yet, there can be no healing process while stress, tension and negativity stand in the way. Does it follow, therefore, that any means we can employ to eliminate these negatives – even quick-fix solutions that have no long-term curative roles – have to be good for us in the long term? I believe so.

To be on the ideological safe side, however, *Instant Calm* has a bet both ways. As well as being crammed with immediate cures, it also devotes a section to the long-term removal of stress, tension and negativity from your life.

So you can expect to find peace not only now, but also in all the days to come.

I did not invent the techniques in this book. Although some have come from disciplines you may not have even heard of, all have been tried and proven by people in addition to myself over the years.

Read *Instant Calm* with an open mind and these techniques will work for you.

STRESS VERSUS CALM

1

THE AGE OF ANXIETY

Notice how your children have stopped worrying about the bomb lately and are growing more and more concerned about the hole in the ozone layer?

Notice how your neighbour's concerns about the spread of AIDS have been replaced by nonspecific concerns about the state of the economy? Notice how many acquaintances are suffering the trauma of marriage breakup? Or financial misfortune?

> By the time you've completed this book, you will know how to eradicate feelings of tension. You will have a whole armoury of soothing techniques that you can employ at any time. You will know fast and effective ways of making yourself feel better – no matter what is going on around you. You will know the 'secret' to being calm.

Think about your own anxieties. Are you growing more peaceful and contented by the day? Or are you feeling progressively more anxious about what's in store?

Look at your work: do you worry about that man who somehow gets the credit for every good thing you do? Or about the supervisor who insists on questioning you about the number of personal telephone calls you make? Or the secretary who refuses to do a thing you ask?

And at home: those ceilings have needed painting for more than two years, the kids insist on the world's most expensive sports shoes, and your husband gets home from work earlier than you yet still expects you to prepare dinner while he watches television programmes about the changing nature of gender roles.

Maybe you work too hard. Not only do you put in too many hours at the office, but you feel guilty about how little time you make available to your family. Maybe you don't work at all; and the harder you try to find employment, the more impossible it seems.

Maybe you've got a short temper, you're overweight, you hate Volvo drivers, or you're just plain crazy.

Maybe you're lonely.

If you're like most people, though, you won't have a single problem that's certain to evoke a note of sympathy . . . only that, from time to time, 'things' get you down.

Welcome to the age of anxiety.

Don't worry, be calm

Just as aspirin takes care of a headache without taking into consideration the fact that you might have drunk too much last night or that you might need glasses, *Instant Calm* is going to take care of those moments of stress, those pangs of angst – with little consideration for the cause. By employing the right techniques, it is possible to make yourself feel better in just a few moments.

You already know this. How many times have you reached for a chocolate bar when you're depressed? Or a cigarette when you're tense? Or turned on the television set when you couldn't face another moment of drama? Those actions did not work for long, of course, but they probably – but only for a moment – made you feel better.

You will find *Instant Calm* infinitely more powerful and satisfying than any of those measures.

By the time you've completed this book, you will know how to eradicate feelings of tension. You will have a whole armoury of soothing techniques that you can employ at any time. You will know fast and effective ways of making yourself feel better – no matter what's going on around you. You will know the 'secrets' of being calm.

Better still, you will know how to become calm – in an instant!

CALM IN AN INSTANT!

'Calm.'

Say it a few times. The mere sound of the word is enough to start you feeling that way.

Imagine how good you would feel if you could go through life feeling totally calm and at ease – no matter what those around you did to test your patience, no matter how much doom and gloom the newspapers preached, no matter where the economy was taking your income or your savings. Wouldn't it be wonderful?

Not only would you cope with life's obstacles much better, but you would appreciate life more. You would enjoy a zest and enthusiasm for living that ordinary people hardly know, and you would look forward to every day with a boundless sense of adventure. Unfortunately, to achieve such a permanent state requires commitment and hard work.

Instant Calm is more about crisis control.

It is about restoring your sense of wellbeing when things go wrong; it is about helping you to feel better when, under normal circumstances, you would be feeling terrible; it is about coping with the trying things that happen in each and every one of our days.

Instant Calm is about crisis control. It is about restoring your sense of wellbeing when things go wrong; it is about helping you to feel better when, under normal circumstances, you would be feeling terrible; it is about coping with the trying things that happen in each and every one of our days.

How calm is that? It will vary from person to person. And, obviously, it will depend on the circumstances you are faced with. But, at the very least, there is one thing you can be certain of ... *you will feel a whole lot better from having used this book*!

How fast is instant?

Go on, admit it, you've been spoiled. For the last forty years the media have been telling you that you never have to wait, that everything worthwhile – from soup to housing loans to shopping nirvana – can be attained in an instant. So as well as living in an age of anxiety, you are living in an age of instant solutions.

Instant Calm has been conceived and researched with brevity in mind. Just like an aspirin, it is intended for fast, albeit temporary, relief from symptoms – the symptoms of stress and anxiety.

Will these 'instant' techniques work in thirty seconds?

In some cases, absolutely. If you do sufficient preparation work many of them will be instantaneous.

If, however, you flick through these pages and never think about their content until a Boeing 747 falls out of the sky and lands on your neighbour's house, you may have to wait just a few minutes for maximum results. You may even have to use a combination of techniques to achieve what you want to achieve – it is not by chance that this book contains such a wide variety of techniques for you to choose from.

While some may be better suited to one person than they are to another, you will find every one has the potential to provide a simple and effective relief from the symptoms of stress. And, when you have mastered combinations of these techniques, you will indeed have powerful skills at your disposal.

Where do they come from?

You may ask how I know about these techniques. Where did they come from? How do I know they will work?

Most have come from natural therapists of one sort or another. Several of them were offered by people I have come in contact during my speaking engagements relating to the Calm Technique. Some are the products of workshops conducted with this very book in mind. And still others are simply common sense.

It would be a great omission if I did not admit there have been sceptics. A significant number of those I consulted denied there was any such thing as quick (or immediate) relief from stressful symptoms.

Indeed, my local MD was adamant that such a thing did not exist – at least not in a non-pharmaceutical form.

He was wrong.

People have been doing it for aeons. When an angry person reaches for the knitting, or storms off for a brisk walk around the block, or punches the wall, or takes three deep breaths and says 'I am not angry, I am not angry, I am not angry', or smiles stupidly when they should be screaming, or bursts into tears – that person is immediately dealing with the symptoms of stress. Moreover, if it weren't for these abilities, I believe the life expectancy of the average Western person would be greatly reduced as a result.

You will find many of the suggestions within these pages will work immediately and profoundly. I cannot nominate which of them will work best for each particular situation – that is a matter of experimentation for you. However, many will have the capacity to revolutionise the way you react to worry, anxiety and nervousness; many will have the capacity to neutralise the problems life throws up; and others will give you the strength to cope with life's most trying situations.

Together, we will ensure this is how *Instant Calm* works for you.

Will it work?

There are more techniques in this book than you will use in a lifetime. Some will work easily for you; others may take a little time to perfect.

Do not be put off by the seemingly esoteric nature of some.

I have spent almost ten years researching and testing these techniques. None are based on hearsay. All have been used and vouched for by others, as well as myself.

A great many of these techniques are being used, time and time again, by suc-

> The power, as well as the limitation, of almost all therapies is what you believe. Or, more correctly, what you allow yourself to believe.

cessful psychologists, stress counsellors and psychotherapists. Whilst some of their therapies may be unconventional, they are not 'mumbo jumbo'.

The power, as well as the limitation, of almost all therapies is what you believe. Or, more correctly, what you allow yourself to believe.

How many people do you know who have capacity to achieve, yet cannot allow themselves to believe they are capable of it? More than likely, you have done so yourself at some time or another. Remember the first time you tried roller skates? If you'd just rolled down the footpath, placing your faith in ballbearings and gravity, chances are you would have gone quite some distance and not fallen at all. But what happened? You started to roll, then your belief system told you were incapable of rolling this well on your first outing, so you landed on your seat. Or had to steady yourself. So the limiting factor in learning to roller skate was not your skill, it was not your athletic prowess, it was your belief.

No matter what the undertaking, if you can suspend your disbelief, you can succeed. Have you read about those self-help courses that culminate with the participants walking barefoot over burning coals? If you can suspend your disbelief, you can succeed in anything.

Before you judge any of the techniques in this book, consider this one fact: the most cynical people in the world also happen to be those who suffer most from stress-related problems.

What does that tell you? Approach this book with an open mind and you will find the answers you are searching for.

Believe it, and you will be calm.

A note to 'Type A' people

As unfashionable as this personality categorisation may be, many of the readers of *Instant Calm* will display what is commonly described as Type A behavioural characteristics. According to the stereotype, Type A people generally suffer more from self-induced stress problems than Type B.

One of the dominant characteristics of Type A behaviour is impatience. The Type A reader will have a tendency to flick through the pages, snatching a few paragraphs here and there, giving them a 30-second trial, then moving on to something else.

To treat the techniques of this book in such a way is simply perpetuating the stress-producing behaviour patterns that Type A people are renowned for.

A second characteristic of Type A people is the belief that they are more in control, and more knowledgeable, than others. Invariably, the

Type A person will look at every *Instant Calm* technique, and see a faster or better way of doing it.

If you are a Type A person, I urge you to give all of the techniques that follow the benefit of the doubt. Consider them in detail. If, after having experimented, you believe there is a better or faster way of applying them, then please experiment.

But taking shortcuts is typical Type A behaviour and often only exacerbates the condition you are trying to relieve.

*Soon, you will be calmer
than you would ever have
believed possible.*

3

HOW TO
MAKE THIS
BOOK WORK
FOR YOU

What can you sensibly expect from using the techniques in this book?

To be frank, I don't believe they're going to ease all your concerns if that Boeing 747 falls out of the sky on to your neighbour's house. Where they *will* have an impact is with those trying, niggling and escalating stresses of your everyday life.

Using techniques from this book, you could reasonably expect to:

- find relief from tension, anxiety and fatigue
- cope better with everyday problems
- be emotionally stronger
- improve your concentration
- be more positive
- be more tolerant
- get more out of life.

Yes, you can expect all of the above. Yes, it is easy to achieve. And yes, you are going to feel better after reading this book. However, the benefits you derive from using the techniques of *Instant Calm* will be in direct proportion to the effort you devote to learning them. This is no different to any other form of training – the more you put into your preparation, the more get out of its usage.

To maximise the benefits, therefore, I urge you to do three things:

- read the whole book
- do sound preparation work
- relax, and have faith in the techniques.

Read the whole book

How you read this book is going to have a great effect on the results you get from it.

You would probably be expecting too much to think that any technique you chose at random from these pages (almost certainly it will be the simplest) will be the one that works best for you. That is not necessarily the case.

To get the maximum benefits, you may need to employ several of these techniques. To do that, you will have to be familiar with many of them; you will need to know how they work *before* you actually need them. Only then can you decide which techniques, and which combinations, work best for you.

Be prepared

Have you ever watched how babies are taught to swim? One of the very first things they learn is orientation: how to get back to the side of the pool. The trainers go over and over this simple technique until the baby does it automatically.

Much later baby learns how to tread water.

Now, if you're a swimmer, you'll know that the very last thing you'll ever need to think about is how to get back to the side of the pool. You do it automatically. Similarly, when you're out of your depth in the sea or in a pool, you begin to tread water – automatically. If you have to stop and think about it, if you have to work out how to do it most effectively once you're in trouble, you're probably on the way to the bottom.

The same applies to overcoming stress.

If you wait until you're really in trouble before thinking through the techniques in this book, you will have forgone their most potent benefits. To get the most from *Instant Calm*, practise the techniques beforehand. Memorise some of them. Learn about breathing. Know how to access these skills – automatically.

Then, when the need arises, you will be able to concentrate on solutions rather than techniques. That is what this book is all about.

Be positive

A positive attitude is the key to this book.

The key to success in anything to do with self-improvement or self-enlightenment – particularly when it applies to the emotions – is the way you approach the solutions.

For these *Instant Calm* techniques to have maximum benefit, you must approach them positively. It is not sufficient for you to want them to work for you – you have to know they're going to work for you.

Because you're going to make them work for you!

Relax. It sounds harder than it is. You will succeed, you will be calm, and you will reject fear and anxiety whenever and however you choose . . . if your approach is positive.

Page after page, I will keep emphasising just how easy it is to go through your days feeling calm and collected. You will be assured that most of the techniques I write about have been used, over and over again, by natural therapists and their clients – and have been found to be extremely effective. By the end of this book you will be convinced that these simple techniques will help you handle stress and crises.

Be patient

See if you recognise this scenario.

You're feeling anxious. Someone tells you there are two ways of dealing with what you're feeling: Technique A, which takes ten minutes to work, or Technique B, which takes eleven.

You start on Technique A but, after only a few minutes of launching yourself into it, impatience gets the better of you. 'This is not working, I'll have to try the other one.' You immediately turn to the alternative, Technique B. But, because you have given neither A nor B your full attention, you succeed with neither.

Most of us are guilty of such impatience at one time or another. The reason is not so hard to understand: restlessness is a classic symptom of stress. The more stressed or anxious you become, the more impatient you become in your search for relief (if that is what you seek). Obviously such an attitude can only be counterproductive.

Be patient when using the techniques in this book. Take your time to get to know them. Take your time when applying them. And if at first attempt they don't work the way you expect them to, take a walk around the block, then come back and have another go.

But, what about ...

Okay, let's get all the doubts out of the way before we go any further. Will these techniques work if that 747 falls out of the sky and lands on your neighbour's house?

That depends on you. By approaching them the right way, you can make these techniques work in any situation. Even disasters. But to get the most from them, keep your expectations in check. Learn to expect the maximum result every time, but learn not to be disappointed if you achieve only 50 per cent effectiveness on some days and 90 on others.

Be comforted by the fact that you have the most thorough book ever compiled on this topic, that you've learned some of the most effective techniques conceived over the past 5000 years, and that you will probably get even better results if you apply them once again in half an hour.

Then be assured that, after all this, you *will* feel better.

The Keys to Using This Book

To get the most from **Instant Calm**, *practise the techniques beforehand. Memorise some of them. Learn about breathing. Know how to access these skills – automatically.*

BE PREPARED

Read how things work beforehand, practise a couple of the techniques you feel most comfortable with, then stay with them. For maximum effectiveness, you may have to combine several.

BE PATIENT

Recognise how stress works. One of its characteristics is restlessness: the moving from one thing to another. Ensure the variety of techniques in this book does not become a stress factor in itself.

BE POSITIVE

Concentrate on the solution, not whether the technique is working or not – that is something to evaluate *after* you've applied it for the desired length of time.

BE PRACTICAL

How much can you reasonably expect from one reading of a book? Expecting too much can be a stress in itself. There are more than a hundred different techniques discussed here; at least some of them are going to work for you. Put your faith in them.

4

CALM CHOICES

Eliminating stress and anxiety from your life is easy. Essentially, you have two choices: you change the circumstances that cause you stress, or you change the way you deal with them.

The first alternative – changing the circumstances that cause you stress – is much easier to write about than it is to achieve. At its most basic, it could be as simple as changing a job that causes you to lose sleep at night. Or leaving a wife who treats you like an unpaid servant. Or getting a court order to prohibit your ex-husband from interfering in the children's education. Or moving to another town where unemployment benefits stretch much further. Or going to another country where your face hasn't been splashed across the pages of the financial press.

> Generally, the most effective way to overcome stress and anxiety is not so much to try to change the situations themselves, but simply to change the way you deal with them.

These are extreme solutions. They are difficult to accomplish and, often, even more stressful than the situations you escaped.

In most instances, the fastest way to overcome stress is not so much to change the situations that cause it, but simply to change the way you deal with them.

You can change yourself

One of the boom industries of the past decade is self-help. Average people of average motivation suddenly found that, with a modicum of guidance, they could transform themselves in ways which their grandparents would never have considered possible.

You may be cynical. But the undeniable fact is it has worked for millions. And it will work for you.

With nothing more than the guidance of this book, you will be able to transform yourself from someone who is a victim of stress and anxiety into someone who is impervious to it, and who is calm and stress-free most of the time (if that is what you desire).

How? Once again, you are faced with two clear-cut choices. Either you change yourself physically, or you change yourself attitudinally.

The ideal is a combination of the two.

Physical change

Unlike the Incredible Hulk, the capacity for changing your physical make-up is limited. Or is it? You can change yourself simply by popping a couple of Valium. Or by downing a bottle of vodka. (Neither of these is recommended, by the way, for dealing with stress and anxiety.)

There are, however, more positive physical changes you can effect to deal with the tensions of modern life.

For a start, you can improve your physical fitness – the fitter you are, the better able to cope you will be.

You can improve your eating and drinking habits. If you doubt the effects that food has on your emotional state – that is, the way you cope with external stressors – try this simple test: spend two days eating heavy protein foods (meat and the like), then two days eating raw fruit and vegetables. On the vegetarian days, you will feel a dramatic improvement in your ability to cope and to relax, nothing is more certain.

Similarly, a day without coffee and alcohol (if you generally indulge in them) will make an equally noticeable difference to the way you feel. On the other hand, if you have an addiction to either of those substances, you will probably not notice the difference.

Even your posture influences the way you handle stress and tension. The person in Figure 1a, overleaf, is less capable of handling pressure than the person in Figure 1b. Why? For a start, the slumped shoulders and dropped neck have the effect of inhibiting the breathing to the upper chest which, in turn, restricts your ability to breathe deeply and relaxedly. But, even more than that, the posture appears defeatist, submissive and weak.

If you ever have any doubt that appearances affect the way you feel try this: walk around the block proudly, chin up, shoulders back, looking people squarely in the eye; then walk around again with your shoulders stooped, head down, feet shuffling. The first walk will leave you with a significantly better feeling than the second.

A great many of the techniques in this book are about physical actions you can take to rid yourself of anxiety as well as to combat the natural tendency many of us have towards becoming anxious.

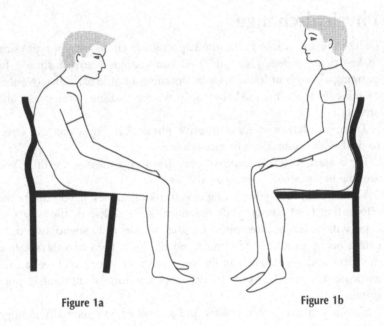

Figure 1a   Figure 1b

Attitudinal change

Contrary to what common sense suggests, it is easier to change bodies than it is to change habits and attitudes.

For the rest of this book we are going to put your negative, stress-encouraging attitudes to the test. You are going to learn new ways to relax, to reject stress and anxiety. You are going to learn ways of dealing with those conditions which cause you to feel tense and irritable. You are going to learn how to reorganise your priorities.

These techniques are going to work, rest assured, just as they have for hundreds of thousands of others just like you.

5

THE CONDITION YOU ARE ABOUT TO OVERCOME

Know your enemy

It used to be 'nerves'. Later, it was referred to as anxiety. These days, almost everyone calls it stress. It is the enemy.

You've probably read those books and articles that urge you to love your stress – unquestionably an attention-getting, and probably a positive, way of getting you to look at a negative condition. The effectiveness of such an attitude, however, varies according to what you call stress.

One model used by stress researcher H. Selye, and featured in *Stress Research: Issues for the Eighties*, highlights four different types of stress.

At one extreme (Figure 2) we have *eustress*, which is the stress that accompanies the exciting things in life – the rollercoaster ride, the first kiss, the lottery win; this is positive stress, something we should all have a little of in our lives. *Under-stress* is the opposite: it accompanies feelings of boredom, hopelessness, physical immobility; it has a negative effect. *Over-stress* is where you push yourself beyond your limits; it can happen as easily in business as it does in marathon races and, again, has a negative effect. *Distress* is the obvious: unresolved frustration, fear, anger, anxiety.

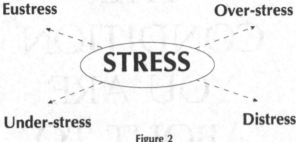

Figure 2

For the purposes of this book, however, I have divided all of these conditions into two categories: positive stress and negative stress. The ideal combination is some positive stress – without it life would be very dull and less effective – with as little of the negative stress as can be achieved.

POSITIVE STRESS	NEGATIVE STRESS
■ Your football team is just about to score.	■ You're late for work, you have an important meeting, and you're stuck in traffic.
■ You race your five-year-old son across the park.	■ You don't know how you're going to afford the rent this month.
■ Your favourite singer is about to appear on stage.	■ You've just had a terrible argument with your girlfriend.
■ You are in the middle of a downhill ski run (and know what you're doing).	■ Your neighbour informs you two policemen were looking for you earlier in the day.
■ That man you've admired for the past year has just asked you to lunch.	■ Your pay cheque bounces.
■ Your best friend has just turned up, unannounced, after three years abroad.	■ You're very worried about your health.

As you can see from the table on the previous page, many stresses are positive. Taken in moderation, they can enrich your life and keep you feeling young and alive.

Studies have shown that individuals who lack positive stress in their life seldom reach peak efficiency. If you look at the graph below you will see how a manageable degree of stress can actually be enriching and performance-enhancing.

It is *negative* stress that is your enemy.

So much for the semantics of stress. The reason you're reading this book, however, is that you are concerned with the debilitating effects of its negative state.

Negative stress is blamed for all sorts of ailments: from the escalating incidence of heart disease, to obesity and hives. It causes hypertension, indigestion, constipation, palpitations, impatience, insomnia and impotence. But, worst of all, it makes you feel lousy.

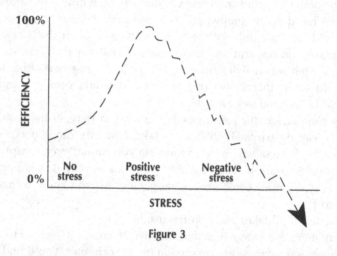

Figure 3

Relax; you won't have to put up with it much longer.

Negative stress works in two ways: it creates immediate problems and discomforts (probably the reason you bought this book in the first place), and causes even more of them in the long term – indeed, it wreaks most damage through the slow accumulation of harmful side effects.

It follows then, that if you overcome the effects of negative stress when it first appears, you will be doing good for yourself in the long term. Hence, used properly, *Instant Calm* will bring profound, long-term benefits to your life.

The enemy within

Pain and misery are very subjective things. Have you ever wondered why boxers don't say 'Ouch', or why footballers break limbs and get bloody gashes, yet continue to watch the remainder of the game from the sideline instead of dashing off to hospital?

Last night, I believed the most painful thing that could happen to a human being was to stub a naked toe against a marble table – it was a pain that increased in direct proportion to the amusement of the onlookers.

One of my acquaintances believes that a broken limb – she broke her wrist – has definite compensations in the pain stakes. Strangers cooed and told her how unlucky she was; she could look at the X-rays and the plaster on her arm and know exactly what her problem was; the ache she felt was real and, most of all, specific to one part of her body; and she knew that sooner or later the cast would come off and she would be as good as new again.

By comparison, the pain caused by intense anxiety, or by doubt and worry, can be extremely difficult to take. Not only can you expect no sympathy from others, most of the time you cannot even accept what is going on yourself. You probably won't know why it is happening; you may not even know *what* is happening. All you know is that you feel bad.

Because it all takes place on the inside.

But there are external manifestations of what's taking place. The more obvious of these are covered in the next chapter. You'll find most of them familiar – even though you may not have thought about, nor even noticed them, in any specific way.

These are the signals from within. Study them. Learn to recognise them for what they are. Because only after you recognise them can you learn how to deal with them.

The physiological process

Unlike most ailments, stress doesn't pass with time. It is self-perpetuating. It builds and builds until it is a major influence on your mind and body, until it dominates almost every action you take, every emotion you feel, and every thought you think.

The reason for this is biological rather than neurotic.

Human beings, like all animals, are biologically equipped for regular episodes of fighting or fleeing. There was a time when this was necessary. Primitive man, when confronted by hostile animal or adversary, had the choice: either stay and fight, or flee for his life. While he was making this decision, his body was preparing for either eventuality. With no conscious effort on his part, his adrenal glands began secreting adrenaline and epinephrine hormones; his muscles tensed, pulse quickened, blood pressure rose, digestion ceased; his breath came more rapidly. In other words, he was perfectly equipped for either fight or flight.

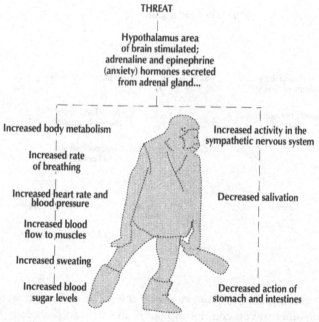

THREAT

Hypothalamus area
of brain stimulated;
adrenaline and epinephrine
(anxiety) hormones secreted
from adrenal gland...

Increased body metabolism

Increased rate
of breathing

Increased heart rate and
blood pressure

Increased blood
flow to muscles

Increased sweating

Increased blood
sugar levels

Increased activity in the
sympathetic nervous system

Decreased salivation

Decreased action of
stomach and intestines

Figure 4

In today's world, every mishap, confrontation, doubt and mistake seems to activate this 'fight or flight' mechanism.

However, the difference between your fight or flight response and primitive man's is what follows it. The primitive man resolved his stressful situation simply by performing one of the options at his disposal: he fought or he fled. Either way, the strenuous effort of his muscles used up the chemicals in his system, whereby he began to calm down and his stress dissolved.

In your case, it's not so simple. When your fight or flight mechanism is activated, you have to remain at your desk. Or behind the wheel of your cab. Or behind the sales counter. And all you can do is *brood*. Your nerves and muscles are all primed for fighting or fleeing, your adrenaline is flowing, and there's nothing you can do about it except brood.

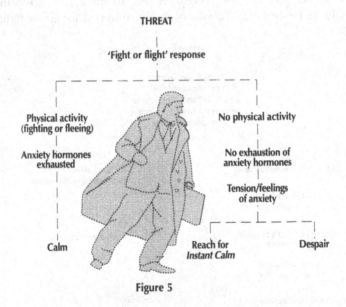

THREAT

'Fight or flight' response

Physical activity
(fighting or fleeing)

Anxiety hormones
exhausted

Calm

No physical activity

No exhaustion of
anxiety hormones

Tension/feelings
of anxiety

Reach for
Instant Calm   Despair

Figure 5

If you could grab your supervisor by the collar and frogmarch her out of the office, if you could jump out of the cab and physically push that offending garbage truck out of your path, or if you could leap across the sales counter and throttle that arrogant customer, you might dispense of some of the stress (though such actions may lead to other, maybe more serious stresses).

But you just can't do these things. You need your job; garbage trucks are not easily pushed out of the way; society does not approve of violent sales assistants. So you're stuck in a passive situation for the rest of the day, with anxiety hormones rampant throughout your bloodstream and your stress levels building and building.

Is it any wonder you've been dying for this book to come out?

6

SIGNALS FROM WITHIN

The fact that you're reading this book is indication enough that you recognise stress for what it is and can do. But do you recognise it as it is happening, or have you become aware of the fact after some other problem has surfaced? Or after you have begun finding it difficult to cope?

One of the wonderful things about your body is the subtle way it communicates what is happening within you. It is sending you powerful signals most of the time – especially when you place yourself in stressful positions. If you haven't noticed this, don't blame your body; it simply means you haven't been paying attention.

One of the wonderful things about your body is the subtle way it communicates what is happening within you. It is sending you powerful signals most of the time – especially when you place yourself in stressful positions. If you haven't noticed this, don't blame your body; it simply means you haven't been paying attention.

I am not referring to the *emotional* side effects of stress such as anger, aggression and irritability. Nor am I referring to the *conditions* stress seems to induce: sleep disorders, overeating, impotence and the like.

This is entirely about physical signals from your body. They fall into five main categories: muscular, headache, expression, posture and breathing.

Muscular

'I'm feeling tense.' Those three words pretty well explain how stress affects your body – or, more precisely, how your body warns you it is being affected by stress. It warns you in the muscles of many different places.

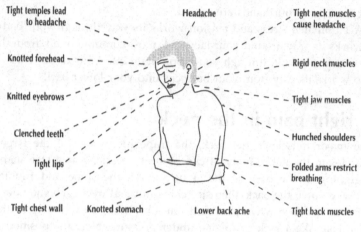

Tight temples lead to headache

Headache

Tight neck muscles cause headache

Knotted forehead

Rigid neck muscles

Knitted eyebrows

Tight jaw muscles

Clenched teeth

Hunched shoulders

Tight lips

Folded arms restrict breathing

Tight chest wall

Knotted stomach

Lower back ache

Tight back muscles

Figure 6

You can feel it in the back of your neck. Tight. Stiff. Restricted. Pulling right up into the back of your head. You can feel it as a tightening of muscles at the base of your cranium (yes, an extension of that tight neck). You probably don't even recognise it as tight muscles, but as a headache. A *tension* headache, people call it; at the back of your head rather than the front. A tight, dull ache rather than the throbbing of a migraine.

You can feel it as a tightening in your shoulders. Down low between your shoulder blades, right across your shoulders and, yes, all the way up to the base of your neck.

You can feel it in your lower back. Ask a masseur or chiropractor where stressed people experience the most problems. The lower back.

You can feel it as a constriction in your chest wall. Tight muscles creating a band-like feeling right across your chest. You fold your arms tightly to compensate. In doing so, you further constrict your breathing, thus adding to the feeling of tension.

You can feel it in your abdominal muscles. A 'scrunched up' feeling, a tight ball around your solar plexus.

You can feel it in your face: jaw clenched tight, forehead pulled down, lips tight.

You can feel it in your fingers. Tight. Clenched. When your hands are clenched, your whole body is preparing itself for action – check it out next time your hands are tensed.

Accumulated stress and tension works its way through your body. It works its way around your face and, most common of all, from the base of your skull, through your shoulders, into your upper back. It also works its way from your buttocks into your lower back.

A right pain in the neck

The major muscle in the neck, the trapezius, is one of the largest muscles in the entire body. It can be best described as a star shape: beginning at the base of the skull, joining the spine and running halfway down the back, then stretching out and over each shoulder.

If you wonder why stress and tension strikes so viciously in this area, just take a look at anyone under pressure. Note the position of the head and shoulders; the entire demeanour is tense. And, more painful still, this tension will remain long after the pressure has passed.

There was a time when this condition served a purpose: it was the combat position so essential to primitive man in his fight or flight state. Today it serves little useful purpose. Left unchecked, it may become nothing more than a pain in the neck. Or worse, a chronic condition.

Getting it in the back

One of today's most common ailments is an extension of this muscular tension – back pain. Chiropractors are thriving. Special pillows, chairs and mattresses are all the rage. Even chains of 'back pain stores', selling everything from neck braces to gravity boots, have appeared.

If you suffer from back problems try this simple test. Next time pain strikes, before you blame your chair, your posture or the idiosyncrasies of your skeleton, take a look at the emotional or other pressures in your life. Usually, you will find they are unbalanced.

The effects of these stresses are even more pronounced if you lead a sedentary lifestyle. More and more medical authorities are accepting that back pain is a by-product of sedentary living – in fact, one lot of research figures I have seen show that more than 80 per cent of all lower back pain is brought about in this way.

How can they all be linked? How can clenched jaw muscles lead to lower back pain? How can a tension headache spring from an aching back? It's all to do with a phenomenon known as referred (or reflex) pain.

Referred pain can cause tension to spread from the skull to the buttocks, from the jaw to the shoulders, in no time at all. The tightness in your neck gradually becomes a tightness in your upper back, gradually becomes a tightness in your lower back, and so on.

> Combine physical inactivity with emotional stress and tension, and you've got neck and back problems.

And because back muscles, even in sedentary people, are extraordinarily strong, they do not transmit pain or spasm, nor suffer wear and tear, as readily as muscles in other parts of the body. Instead, they contract and become progressively tighter, which not only encourages pain in other muscles but, left untreated, can continue until the condition is chronic and your whole skeleton is distorted.

Headache

Although it is most often caused by musculature complications, headache is such a common ailment that it could easily command a book of its own.

Whether we profess to be affected by negative stress or not, most of us are familiar with the 'tension headache', by far the most common of all headache types, and caused by muscular contraction.

Varying in discomfort and intensity, the tension headache generally appears as a dull, throbbing tightness stretching from the back of the neck to the crown of the head, sometimes extending as far as the forehead and temples. Occasionally it is accompanied by nausea-like sensations and dizziness. Unless treated, it can continue for uncomfortable periods of time – or at least until the pressure is relieved.

However the condition is as easy to understand as it is to treat. The

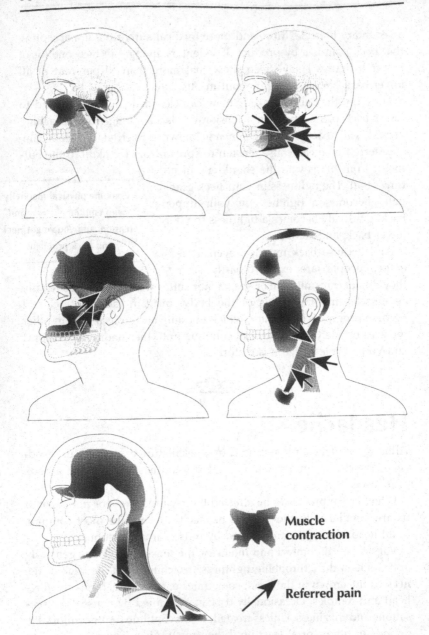

Figure 7

pain stems from muscular contraction or cramp, which can be triggered by simple physical conditions as varied as eyestrain, spinal irregularity, mal-alignment of the bite, or going to sleep with the neck on an awkward angle.

Most often, though, it is triggered by conditions we normally associate with stress and tension.

The first manifestation of your stress may be almost unnoticeable to you – a worried frown, a clamped jaw, or hunched shoulders. But the *extensions* of that condition, the muscle contraction inching along the trapezius muscle in your back, up the back of your neck, cramping your jaw's masseter muscle, tightening around the base of your skull, over your head . . . tighter . . . throbbing . . .

Yes, this is referred pain. You can see in Figure 7 how contractions in various muscle groups 'refer' or trigger pain in other areas. The most common areas of referred pain are around the neck and upper back, closely followed by the buttocks and lower back.

By the end of this book you will know how to deal with bothersome reactions such as these. By the end of this book, you will be an expert at dealing with all kinds of tension.

Posture

Now that you have an idea of how stress effects your musculature, you are probably beginning to get the picture of how it might have an effect on your posture.

Take a look at a person under stress.

The hunched shoulders, bowed head, folded arms – what do they suggest? Tightened muscles across the shoulders, perhaps? Contracting muscles in the back of the neck? And in the chest wall and stomach area, as well?

Look closer. Note the clenched fingers. If you were to look closer still, you would see crossed ankles as well. All these reflect muscle groups that tend to contract during stressful situations. As you can

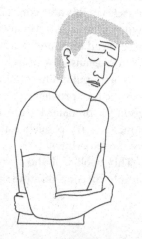

Figure 8

see, muscles play as big a role in your posture as they do in your body language.

By the time you have finished this book, you will know a variety of ways of altering your posture in order to find quick relief from the effects of negative stress.

Expression

Other parts of the body react to negative stress in a similar way to your posture and body language.

The very expression on your face is a reflection of this process. The knotted eyebrows, the furrowed brow, clenched jaw, pursed lips: these are all examples of the way muscles – in this case, facial muscles – react to negative stress. Because they are so visible, and because they have such a pronounced effect on the way you appear and feel, they deserve a category all of their own.

The most visible muscular area where stress manifests is the forehead. The frown and the tightened eyebrows are clear indications of the sufferer's frame of mind. You can actually feel your stress concentrating in these areas.

A less visible area of tension, but one which can cause even more painful side effects, is the upper jaw. Next time you feel angry, or anxious, or worried, take note of the tightness in your jaw. As the muscles in this area contract, you clench your teeth and this encourages two additional effects: an overall feeling of tightness in your shoulder/ neck/head area, and headache.

Worse, tense jaw muscles have a habit of 'referring' their discomfort. It is a popular line of thought amongst some therapists that many chronic *back* problems stem from the jaw area. I once heard a midwife giving a prenatal lecture insist: 'Tight jaw, tight pelvic floor. If you doubt me, try passing water while you have your jaw clenched'. Feel free to experiment.

This book will show you how to find real calm in no time at all, simply by concentrating on relaxing those expressions.

Breathing

Of all the physical signals your body sends that you're succumbing to the ravages of negative stress, the most critical, the most noticeable, and yet the *least* visible of them all, are the changes in your breathing.

Of all the techniques that follow, the one that will produce the most pronounced and most immediate benefits is the one based on breathing patterns.

The breathing pattern of someone under stress – be it positive or negative stress – is shallow and rapid. This is what you'd expect from a speeded-up heart and pulse rate. Conversely, the breathing pattern of someone in a contented and relaxed state is invariably deep and slow – the reverse of the stressful pattern.

Of all the techniques to follow, the one that will produce the most pronounced and most immediate benefits is the one based on breathing patterns. Use the breath-control techniques in this book and you are well on the way to becoming calm.

Other Signals

Other signals your body sends during moments of stress are less visible than those already covered, but you will still be aware of them.

For many, palpitations are as familiar a response to stress as the tension headache. While these affect people with varying degrees of seriousness, they are still a sign that you may not be handling things as efficiently as you might. Similarly, stomach upsets, sleeping problems, impotence, reduced sex drive, high blood pressure, even major conditions such as heart attack and stroke, are undeniable signs that you are not coping with the stresses of your everyday life.

By the end of this book, you will both recognise these signals and be able to use them to cope with practically anything.

7

SIGNALS FROM THE OUTSIDE

Because they tend to affect you in visible and attention-getting ways, the physical manifestations of negative stress are easy to identify. Behavioural and emotional manifestations, however, are more subtle. Indeed, when these characteristics are pointed out, the sufferer will often disagree that it is stress which causes them.

Let's see if you can recognise these characteristics.

The patterns of your speech

Notice how fast the words come when a child comes running home, pleading to be allowed to go skating with the kids from next door? Or when you hear someone describing a bank robbery she has just witnessed? Or when your husband gets angry about the way you spent all night speaking to that handsome young actor at the party?

You react in a similar way when you're under pressure or suffering from negative stress. Words come quickly. The rhythm of your speech speeds up. Spaces between words are shortened.

Some of the techniques that follow will show you how, simply by varying these very natural characteristics, you will control the condition that causes them. You will well be on the way to calm.

The way you approach activities

How did you go about your work the last time you were 'in a state'? Concentration was difficult; you could only really pay attention to the immediate things you had to do, not the bigger picture or the long-term issues.

If you responded true to type, you probably went to considerable lengths to distract yourself – anything but focus on the tasks at hand. You may even have attempted to perform several different tasks at the one time – succeeding in none, of course, and only exacerbating your 'state'. Yet, in spite of your need for distraction, you would have been greatly irritated if someone had come along and disturbed you.

Negative stress affects people in strange and seemingly illogical ways.

Your attitudes

Not surprisingly, the attitudes of the anxiety-ridden person almost always head towards the negative. While common sense may tell you that negative thinking only worsens the state, usually you are in no frame of mind to alter the course of your thoughts once you are committed to them.

As a result, things appear progressively more gloomy, you become more and more anxious, and until something comes along to break the pattern, you are stuck on an stress spiral.

You make mistakes. You become increasingly impatient. You grow bored (which, in turn, creates stresses of its own). You can

HOW STRESS AFFECTS YOU PHYSICALLY

- Headaches
- Butterflies in the stomach
- Palpitations
- Chest pain
- Skin rashes
- Breathing difficulties
- Diarrhoea
- Constipation
- Reduced sex drive
- Indigestion
- Sleeping difficulties
- Tiredness
- Drug or alcohol abuse
- Speeded-up conversation
- Overeating
- Loss of appetite
- Poor memory
- Dry mouth
- Inability to concentrate
- Over-reaction to events
- Trembling hands
- Cold hands
- Fidgeting
- Grinding teeth

see only the bad side of your self, your surroundings, your condition and the people around you. You compare yourself unfavourably with others. And you are certain that others can only see the bad side of you.

You worry unnecessarily about everything – you over-generalise. You're obsessive. You set unreasonable challenges for yourself, striving to achieve things you really do not believe you can achieve. And with each passing moment, you find it harder to cope.

You are scared.

Negative thinking is the most damaging by-product of negative stress. By learning to overcome one – which you will by the end of this book – you will have learned to overcome the other.

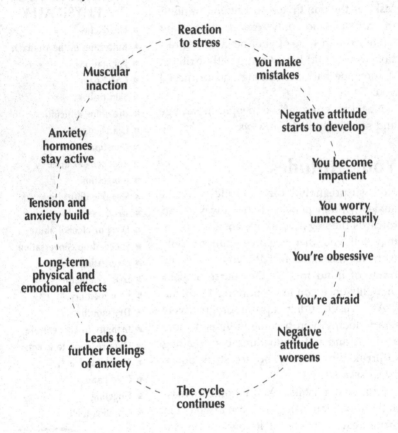

The habits you adopt

Does negative stress cause bad habits?

Ask that question of a smoker and they will have no doubt at all. 'When I'm stressed I have to reach for a cigarette.' *Ergo*, stress perpetuates the smoking habit.

The more accurate perspective, however, is the reverse: bad habits induce negative stress. The more you smoke (to continue the analogy), the more pronounced will be your stress. The more you indulge your addiction, the more you suffer the physiological downsides that accompany it.

(Of course, what's a 'bad' habit to one person may not be to another. Every smoker who reads this will take comfort when I say that some smokers are not victims of their habit and are, therefore, not causing themselves additional stress by smoking. Unfortunately, if you did fit that category, you would not be reading this book . . .)

The 'bad' habits of the stress-affected will be familiar to you. In extreme cases, they smoke too much, drink more coffee than you would consider healthy, seem overly fond of alcohol, and often have a need for tranquillisers or sleeping pills.

Look at the fingers: nervous, twitching, fiddling, drumming on the table in moments of pressure. Look at the creased forehead and the clenched jaw.

I wish I could tell you this book was going to cure you of your smoking habit, or wean you from excessive alcohol. Obviously this will not be the case. What it will do, however, is show you how to adopt new habits. Powerful, life-changing new habits that will have a calming and positive influence on your life. And this, in turn, will make it easier for you to shed any habit you choose.

8

THE CAUSES
OF STRESS

Defining the *symptoms* of negative stress is relatively easy because they are characteristics easily recognised in yourself or others. Defining what *causes* negative stress is another matter entirely.

I have read innumerable books on this topic. Most are convinced that they contain the definitive reasons why people feel anxious and stressed every day; these range from the commonplace (such as an inability to be assertive) through to the exotic (such as an excess of positive ions in the atmosphere).

THE WAYS STRESS AFFECTS YOUR BEHAVIOUR

- Irritability
- Irrationality
- Intolerance of people
- Low tolerance of noise
- Suspiciousness
- Easily bored
- Varying emotional states
- Inability to concentrate
- Pessimism
- Negative attitudes
- Feeling that something is about to go wrong

If you've ever bothered to scan the publications on this topic, you'll find many of them rely on a certain Life Events Scale compiled by two well-known American psychiatrists, Drs Holmes and Rahe. Their stress index provides a numeric stress rating for the common misfortunes in life – for example, it rates Death of a Spouse at 100, and Christmas at a mere 12.

If only all our stress and anxieties could be that formularised!

What rating would we give to feeling jealous about a lover? Or being rejected? Or about feeling lonely or unwanted? Would concern about your job security rate higher or lower on the stress index than Christmas? Does it really matter?

The great majority of people who suffer from negative stress or tension find it impossible to pinpoint the reasons for their anxieties. Even though they may suffer none of the conditions mentioned in that Holmes and Rahe Life Events Scale, nor perhaps any definable condition at all, they are still stressed.

So much the better if you know the exact cause of your stress – that it comes from an insensitive, patronising boss, or from forgetting to pay your telephone bill, or from being caught in the traffic when you're supposed to be meeting someone outside Town Hall – because when you know the cause, you can do something about it.

> Often, stress is the result of conflict within an individual. The forms of such conflict will usually arise from: the desire for intimacy versus the desire for isolation; the desire for independence versus the need for dependence; the desire to compete versus the desire to co-operate; the desire to be impulsive versus the restrictions of social standards.

I have more sympathy for the sufferer who does not know the reason for his or her anxieties.

Yet, this is the most common condition of them all. Most sufferers will tell you their worries and anxieties are the non-specific variety – where they simply feel stressed and tense, and probably have no idea why they're feeling that way at all. They just feel stressed.

If you fit this category, let's see if we can make you feel better by defining the root causes of this 'ill-defined' or 'non-specific' stress.

The Root of All Stress

Invariably, stressors fall into one of three categories: physical, psychological (emotional) or lifestyle-related (behavioural).

Physical stressors can range from illness or violence, to environmental conditions such as extreme cold, hard beds and noisy neighbours. Lifestyle stressors (which are really a combination of physical and emotional conditions) range from high-pressure occupations or poor sleeping habits, to drug and alcohol abuse. Emotional stressors, which are those that originate in your mind, are the most insidious and complex package of them all.

Following are some of the most common root causes of stress and anxiety. You will note that all of these are non-physical, because most stress is the result of what happens inside your head, rather than what happens to your body.

Later in *Instant Calm* you will learn how, by recognising these causes, you can short circuit them, thus inducing calm when and as you desire it.

Anxiety

Although anxiety is a 'result' rather than a 'cause', it is worthy of closer examination. Anxiety is always related to concerns about time, or more specifically, about the future. Whether these are for the foreseeable future – say 30 minutes ahead – or for the distant future, is irrelevant; the fact is they're concerns about something that is only an abstract concept, something that does not exist. Our efforts to bestow on it some form of reality (even in our choice of words like 'foreseeable future' and 'distant future'), along with our efforts to treat the future as something that can be controlled or manipulated, are what create anxiety.

> Most stress and anxiety is the result of what happens *inside your head*, rather than what happens to your body. Frequently, it is also the result of conflict you may be experiencing, even if you don't immediately recognise this.

Guilt

Guilt generally falls into two categories.

a Guilt associated with what you think of yourself – it may be to do with the type of person you are, the attitudes you have, the things you've done, the things you intend doing, or simply things about yourself that you've been conditioned to think are bad or unattractive.

b Guilt associated with what others try to make you feel or do – such as being responsible for their moods or conditions, or making you feel guilty about working late at the office, or spending money on yourself.

Whether inspired by yourself or by others, carrying around feelings of guilt is a major cause of stress.

Deadlines

Set yourself a deadline, or have one set for you, and you are flirting with stress. Take a look at any deadline-oriented occupation, or any deadline-oriented person, and you will often see a hotbed of stress-related problems. The reasons should be obvious: as the deadline nears, and the task demands completion, tensions rise.

Boredom

Is boredom the result of stress, or is it the other way around?

You'll be pleased to know it doesn't really matter, because boredom has to be dealt with if you're to reduce the effects of negative stress in your life. You'll also be pleased to learn that this is one of the stressors most easily overcome.

Vanity

'But I'm not vain,' you protest. This may be so. Yet so much stress is caused not by what you think of yourself, but by what you believe other people may think of you.

How stressful is it when you discover someone else thinks you're vulgar, or dishonest, or naive?

The impact of stressful situations is governed by three factors: being able to predict the stressful event and its outcome; being able to exert some control over it; and having the emotional support of others in the face of these events.

How much anxiety do you feel when people accuse you of being a bad mother, an unprofessional employee, an unreliable friend or a cheat?

Ambition

In many ways, ambition goes hand in hand with deadlines. You have to achieve something within a certain time frame, and you cannot excuse yourself for not reaching this objective.

The fact that you are driven to achieve certain goals need not be a stressor in itself; indeed, some people are invigorated by the challenge. But if your goals are poorly defined – 'I want to be rich', 'I want to be powerful', 'I want to be famous' – or if they are beyond your reach, or beyond the time limit you have set for yourself, expect to feel under pressure.

Frustration

You're caught in heavy traffic on the way to an important meeting, stuck in the lift, cornered by the world's greatest bore, attempting to thread a needle with an invisible eye, desperate to be heard by the head of your department – in themselves, these issues may be relatively minor and everyday inconveniences but, to many of us, they are the pinnacles of frustration.

Frustration leads to negative stress.

Conversely, the greater your fundamental stress level, the greater will be your disposition to become frustrated. Treat one and you treat the other.

Fear

Fear is much the most damaging emotional stressor of them all. You fear that your boyfriend is seeing another woman. You fear that the Tax Department is going to hound you for your very last cent. You fear that the comment you made in the lunch room is going to get back to the boss. You fear that ecological insensitivity is soon going to destroy the planet.

In the great majority of cases, these fears will be centred on something that is not actually happening at the moment and probably will never happen at all. Your fear is that it *may* happen. In more extreme cases, you may not have any idea of what specific issue is causing your fear – you just know that you are feeling uneasy, afraid that something might happen.

With emotions performing as illogically as that, is it any wonder a person feels stressed?

Lust

If you link greed and envy with lust, you end up with a devastating – though possibly entertaining – trio of negative stressors.

For many, lust is a powerful motivator. It has the capacity to soften logic and to blind normally well-balanced people to extremes of folly, insensitivity and self-destructiveness. However, as with ambition, lust is often accompanied by high levels of expectation (a cause of stress) which, in turn, can lead to frustration (another cause of stress) if left unfulfilled.

9

THE
CONDITIONS
OF CALM

To a stressed, anxious or frightened person, a state of calm can be the most desirable, yet the most elusive, of all goals. At the moment of your greatest need it will appear singularly unattainable. Even the process of trying to achieve it will add to your frustration, often exacerbating the original condition.

Yet becoming calm is relatively easy to achieve – if you know how.

Think back on the times of your life when you were in a perfectly calm state. What were you doing? What were the conditions that surrounded you? What was your state of mind?

Instead of coffee, have a glass of water. Or a herbal tea.
Instead of a cigarette, apply one of the techniques that follow. Instead of turning on the radio or television, take comfort in the silence.
Instead of throwing yourself into the nearest group or conversation,
take a couple of minutes outdoors to slow down.

Invariably, those times of peace and tranquillity would have the following attributes in common: Comfort, fresh Air, and Lack of stimuli. If you add one more attribute, Motivation, you have a powerful combination (as well as a convenient acronym) for combating stress.

These are the *conditions* of calm.

Comfort

One of the greatest obstacles to relaxing, yet the one that is most often overlooked when seeking calm, is physical discomfort: uncomfortable temperatures, unnatural seating or resting arrangements and restrictive clothing. Fortunately, most of these conditions are easily remedied.

The ideal room temperature for relaxation is just *slightly warmer* than what is generally considered the most comfortable room temperature (20°C or 68°F). For most people, a degree or so warmer than that is perfect. Of course, if you've just come in out of a heatwave, the ideal temperature may be a degree or so cooler than that.

The next comfort ideal relates to where you sit or rest as you're trying to relax. In these instances, it is not so much that you find comfort, but that you avoid discomfort. For example, a simple, straight-backed chair is an ideal relaxing place for most people (though they may not appreciate this) yet it does not satisfy the conventional notion of a 'comfortable chair'.

The last comfort ideal is the one that will have the most pronounced and immediate effect. It is to do with your clothing. Try the following (where appropriate) and you will immediately begin to feel more relaxed: remove your shoes; undo your tie or neck button; loosen your belt; unclasp your bra strap; slip into 'something more comfortable'.

Air

Have you ever wondered why you feel more calm in the country than you do in the city?

You might be inclined to put it down to the absence of noise. Yet you can sit on a deserted beach, surrounded by the thunderous roar of a heavy surf, and still find a deep state of calm.

It is because of the space and the fresh air.

This is why it is more relaxing to walk down a country road than it is through a deserted (soundless) suburban street. Why it's more relaxing to sail in the wide open sea than it is on a busy harbour. Why a desk next to a window is more relaxing than a desk near the inner wall.

Fresh air is one of the most powerful counterbalances to stress and anxiety. Whether it's wide open space in the outdoors, or a chair placed by an open window, fresh air is at the root of many relaxation techniques.

It is one of the important steps to calm.

Lack of stimuli

City cynics will often decry the 'boring', non-social activities I am recommending as the antithesis of relaxation. They say, for them, relaxation comes from being stimulated – not from being surrounded by space or silence. I hear such comments almost every time the topic of relaxation is brought up.

These opinions sound about as valid and as convincing as the smoker who claims cigarettes are relaxing (I can show you a truckload of physiological evidence to prove the opposite), or as the coffee drinker who claims that a strong coffee soothes the nerves.

Instant Calm is not concerned with your nicotine habits or your coffee consumption. My purpose in mentioning them is simply to point out the fact that they are stimulants and, as such, *excite* the nervous system rather than relaxing it. The same applies for alcohol, marijuana, rock and roll, speeding cars, sweets – I'm sure you can think of a hundred more.

If you need to relax, if you need a fast dose of calm, avoid stimulants. Instead of coffee, have a glass of water. Or a herbal tea. Instead of a cigarette, apply one of the techniques that follow. Instead of turning on the radio or television, take comfort in the silence. Instead of throwing yourself into the nearest conversation, take a couple of minutes outdoors to slow down.

This lack of stimuli – at least for the time you are working at finding calm – is an essential counterbalance to stress and anxiety. It is essential to almost all relaxation and meditation techniques.

Silence

The severely stressed and the anxious avoid it with passion. They claim, and often believe, that silence actually adds to their stress levels. 'I need the radio to relax.'

You should not be fooled by this.

Stress, like most addictions, is deceitful. Just as a cigarette addiction will convince you that you need a cigarette to relax (when you know the opposite is true), and a coffee addiction will convince you that you need an espresso coffee to unwind, your stressful state will try to convince that noise is part and parcel of the relaxation process. It may even convince you that silence is, in itself, stressful.

Hence the stressed person avoids silence at all costs, keeping the radio playing whenever possible, engaging in meaningless chatter simply to avoid that gaping hole in the sound levels.

If you want to be peaceful, if you want to relax, go searching for silence. Absorb it, immerse yourself in it, hang on to it as long as possible. Because in silence can you achieve real calm.

> **If you want to be peaceful, if you want to relax, go searching for silence. Absorb it, immerse yourself in it, hang on to it as long as possible.**

You've no doubt heard of that popular piece of relaxation technology, the float tank. Enthusiasts boast of the blissful state of calm they achieve simply by climbing inside a light-proof tank and floating in a saline solution – in complete silence. It works extraordinarily well, providing relief from the build-ups of everyday stress. Unfortunately you can't carry a float tank around with you.

Go and take a pew in an empty church or temple one day. Sit there a few moments and meditate (that is, sit there and try not to think about anything in particular). Absorb the atmosphere of absolute peace and calm that permeates. Unless you have any strong anti-religious feelings, you will feel relaxed in a very short time. Is it some sort of spiritual energy that achieves this? Is it an air of otherworldliness that allows you to feel this way? For the most part, it will be the silence.

Silence – especially when used creatively – is one of the most powerful counterbalances to stress and anxiety.

Silence is at the root of most relaxation and meditation techniques. (Yes, I know many meditation techniques are based on sounds. But generally these are repeated sounds which, in effect, become hypnotic drones not far removed from silence.) Silence is only a few short steps away from calm.

Silence is at the root of most of the techniques that appear in this book.

Motivation

If you're feeling particularly anxious or stressed, you can be in the quietest place on earth, you can be as comfortable as is humanly possible, you can be totally free of stimulants, and still not achieve what you really want.

To become calm, you have to work at it. You have to be motivated, actively to seek it. This is positiveness at work. The more positive you are that you can achieve something, the more certain you are to be able to do so.

You *can* shrug off the negative effects of stress and anxiety with a minimum of effort. You can be completely relaxed in conditions you never believed you'd be able to cope with. You can even be a calm influence in the lives of all those around you.

You may not have noticed, but you are already a fair way down that path. At this very moment you are much closer to peace and calm – whenever you want it – than most.

How? You have been reading this book.

The Conditions that Lead to Calm

COMFORT

Comfort in environment, in seating and in clothing is a fast and easy way to start to feeling more relaxed. The ideals: a warm place, a straight-backed chair, loosened clothes and no shoes.

AIR

Fresh air tends to reduce much of the pressure when you're feeling stressed or anxious. A stroll in the park will bring more relief than standing shoulder-to-shoulder in a movie queue; a chair by the window will bring more relief than one crammed between others.

LACK OF STIMULI

Lack of stimuli prevents the excitation of your nervous system. Stressful states of mind often lead you to believe certain stimulants are necessary to your relaxation – but who wants to trust stressful states of mind?

Silence (or a sense of silence) is one of the most powerful counterbalances to stress and anxiety. Almost all relaxation and meditation techniques insist on it. Wherever possible, seek calm in silence.

MOTIVATION

Motivation is the most important element of all. As much as you would like external agents to do it all for you, the only way to find a real state of calm is to assume the responsibility and to go after it yourself.

INSTANT CALM:

the techniques

IN CASE OF EMERGENCY

As you would expect, my advice for getting the most out of *Instant Calm* is not to try any of the techniques that follow until you've read the whole book.

If you are a person under stress, however, it is unlikely you will listen to this wisdom. Impatience is the hallmark of the stress-affected person.

So what do you do in the case of an emergency?

What are you meant to do if you've just barged into the book-shop in a flap, seized this book because of the promise of its cover, then flicked through until you came to this page?

Simple.

Just read through the section on breathing, then turn to pages 70–2 and follow the guidelines there. Within minutes you should be feeling more powerful and in control.

10

REVERSING NEGATIVES

One of the over-riding principles of *Instant Calm* is that the harmful effects of negative stress can be overcome – at least temporarily – simply by reversing the physical, emotional or physiological symptoms that cause them. While this may not be the epitome of holistic principles, it does work beautifully. And isn't that all you should expect from a book that promises instant cures?

Many of the following techniques are little more than reversals of conditions that cause or are caused by negative stress. If, for example, you know that tight jaw muscles can lead to a tension headache, then you simply slacken the jaw muscles. And, guess what! The tension headache begins to ease. Yes, it can be as easy as that. (How you go about effectively slackening the jaw muscles, though, is another matter.)

Many of the causes of negative stress are lifestyle related. Can complex lifestyle factors or events be countered by simple, easy-to-use techniques? As glib and simplistic as it may sound, the most effective way of avoiding the ill-effects of a high-stress lifestyle is by adopting a low-stress one. Or at least the characteristics of one.

Elementary? Maybe. But don't mistake simplicity for ineffectiveness. Simple as they may be, these solutions are extraordinarily effective.

Please remember that, even though some of these solutions may appear obvious, *they work*. Whether they work individually or in combination is a matter for experiment. However they do work. And if you approach them positively they will work for you.

For convenience, I have divided these techniques into some of their better known categories. These are the Calm Routes.

The Calm Routes

Ridding yourself of stress and becoming calm can happen in four fundamental ways: spiritually, emotionally, intellectually and physically.

The techniques of *Instant Calm* concentrate on the latter three. Once you have got those three areas in order, the remaining route – the spiritual – happens naturally (if that's what you want to happen).

Using all four of these routes in combination is what holistic stress relief is all about.

The spiritual route

Whilst not the focus of this book, this is considered by many to be the most profound and surest way of finding true calm.

The emotional route

For many personality types, there is no other way to calm: stress is caused by emotional factors, stress can only be countered by emotional means. This book contains many such means, with techniques appealing to the conscious as well as the subconscious mind.

The intellectual route

One has to ask: 'How can an intelligent, reasoning person become a victim of such an illogical thing as stress?' This book recognises that many of us – particularly those who would wade through a book of this size – are governed by the intellect. For this reason, many of the techniques that follow are designed to appeal in this way.

The physical route

This is the most basic route of them all, and perhaps the most demonstrably beneficial. It involves techniques that range from acupressure, to massage, to diet, and to physical objects that relieve stress.

11

THE BREATH OF LIFE

Whether you notice it consciously or not, one of the first things you observe about a stressed, nervous person is their breathing pattern. And the rhythms of their speech.

A stressed, nervous person breathes in shallow, rapid breaths. His or her speech is faster, more frenetic than usual. If you enter into conversation with such a person, you will begin to match these patterns – your breathing will start to become more shallow and rapid, the rhythm of your speech will speed up to match theirs. (This common psychological phenomenon is called 'pacing' and is the reason why you should avoid stressed people if you want to stay calm.)

Shallow breathing reduces the level of carbon dioxide in your bloodstream. When this level drops too low, it causes a constriction of the blood vessels throughout the body. This, in turn, reduces oxygen to the brain – often by more than 20 per cent – which promotes dizziness, feelings of tension and headache.

> By being able to control your breathing, by harnessing this incredibly powerful life force, you can control the way you feel. You can find calm in moments of stress. You can easily cope with almost any pressure.

Now, what are the characteristics of a calm, relaxed person?

His/her breathing is slow and deep – almost lazy. His/her speech patterns are slow and relaxed.

If you are in a state of stress or anxiety and are confronted by someone who is completely relaxed, you will find these patterns irritating. (You'll probably rationalise it in some impatient way – 'I don't have time for small talk', or something like that.) Think back to how people in an office behave when one of their group returns from four weeks' vacation and tries

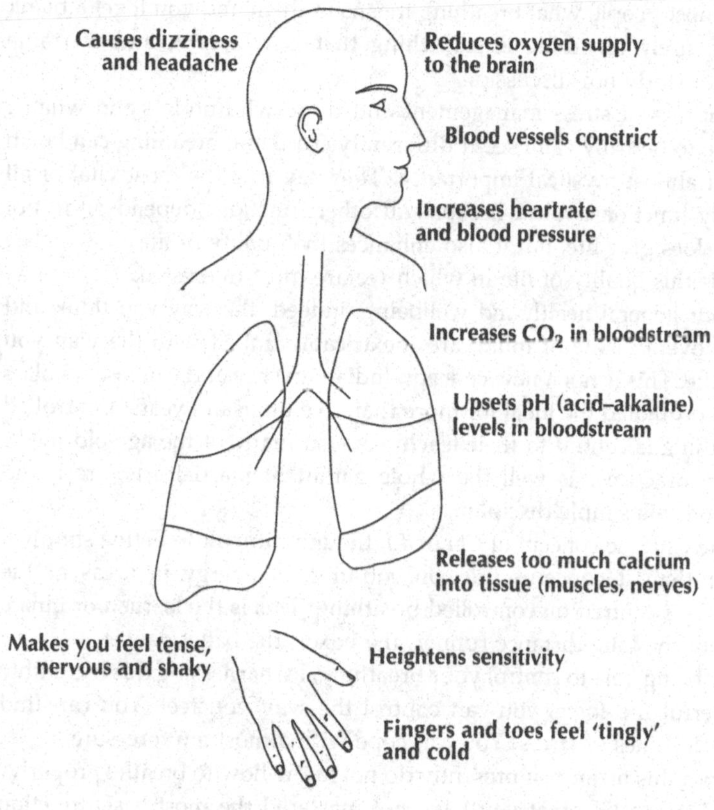

Causes dizziness
and headache

Reduces oxygen supply
to the brain

Blood vessels constrict

Increases heartrate
and blood pressure

Increases CO_2 in bloodstream

Upsets pH (acid–alkaline)
levels in bloodstream

Releases too much calcium
into tissue (muscles, nerves)

Makes you feel tense,
nervous and shaky

Heightens sensitivity

Fingers and toes feel 'tingly'
and cold

Figure 9
The physical effects of shallow breathing

to catch up on business. Often, that person's slowed speech and breathing rhythms will actually aggravate the stressed people in the group. Look around you, you'll see it happening all the time.

Whether you're aware of it or not, the way you breathe has an enormous influence on the way you feel. This is particularly true when it comes to feeling calm and relaxed.

5000 years of breathing

Ask most people what breathing means to them and you'll get a blank look; surely breathing is something that just *happens*, and warrants neither study nor discussion.

Students of stress management and those who understand what it is like to be truly calm see it differently. To them, breathing can be an act of almost mystical importance. They say it is the most vital of all bodily functions. Why? Because all other functions depend on it; not only does give life, but it also enhances the quality of life.

It is this quality of life in which we are most interested.

Your general health and wellbeing, indeed, the way you think and your overall state of mind, are inextricably linked with the way you breathe. This is not a new concept. Indian mystics and Chinese scholars have promoted the ideal for more than five thousand years. Controlled breathing is central to their teachings – so many of the age-old medi-tation practices, as well the whole gamut of martial arts, are based around this simple discipline.

The Chinese concept of *Chi* or *Ki*, though difficult to define simply – other than it concerns the concentration of energy in areas of the body – is centred on controlled breathing. This is the learned or innate skill of the long-distance runner, the boxer, the ballet dancer.

By being able to control your breathing, by harnessing this incredibly powerful life force, you can control the way you feel. You can find calm in times of stress. You can cope with almost any pressure.

Does this mean you presently do not know how to breathe properly? Am I suggesting that you have not mastered the most basic function of your entire being?

I'm afraid that's exactly what I'm suggesting.

Learn to breathe again

Almost every body you look at today has lent itself to 'bad' breathing habits: stooped shoulders, constricted throats and chests, shallow breaths. This is so prevalent it is considered normal.

Would you believe that a great many aspects of your life would improve – sometimes dramatically – if you knew how to breathe prop-erly? It's true. Not only will your body be more relaxed and healthier, but your emotions and state of mind will be as well.

Breathing is unique among all human functions in that it is the only involuntary activity of the body that we have conscious control over. Being able to do it is one thing; being able to do it properly is quite something else.

No one knows better than I how difficult it is to excite people about this activity. But even though you may find it difficult to accept at first, one of the most profound life-changing skills you are going to take from this book is learning how to breathe properly. This, in turn, will provide you with an exquisitely simple shortcut to feeling calm.

Learning to breathe properly is easy; you will master it in minutes. Learning to breathe this way *all the time*, however, takes effort. And concentration.

Before we examine the techniques involved in proper breathing, it is necessary to look at the physiology of breathing. And that begins with lungs.

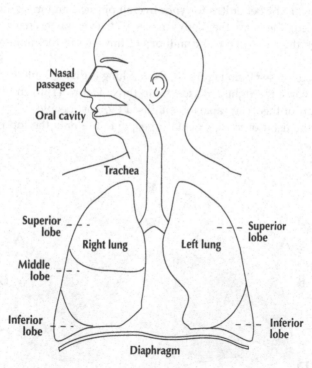

Figure 10

The wonder of lungs

Correct breathing is not simply about getting air into your lungs and then getting it back out again. Ideally, your intake of air will be equal to the capacity of your lungs.

Deep breathing of this nature is a cleansing and holistic experience. Once you have savoured it, you will be astounded at how profound and energising it can be.

Yet the average person seldom does this. Most of the time they use only a fraction of their total lung capacity and, even when consciously trying to breathe deeply, are incapable of doing so.

To understand why this is so, it is necessary to have a basic under-standing of the function and anatomy of this amazing organ, the lungs. The fundamental purpose of lungs is to introduce oxygen to, and to remove carbon dioxide from, the bloodstream; the more oxygen they can deliver, the better it is for your overall physical and mental health. Simplified, the way the body manages this is by exchanging air between the atmosphere and millions of tiny sacs in the lungs known as alveoli.

As you can see from Figure 10, the left lung is divided into two parts (lobes) while the right is divided into three. Figure 11 illustrates how only part of this lung capacity is utilised by most people.

It is the habit of most sedentary people to use only the top portion

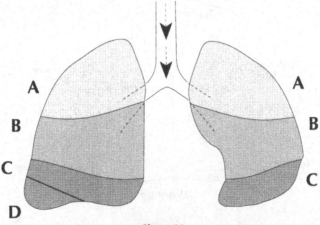

Figure 11

(A), the superior lobe of each lung. They breathe often and there is little or no expansion of the chest wall when they do so. Shallow breathing of this type is not only inefficient, but fails to expose the major volume of the lungs to fresh air.

More common, especially amongst fitter folk, is 'middle breathing' where more of the lung capacity (B) is accessed. In this instance, contracting intercostal muscles move the ribs upward and outward, allowing more air into the lungs. Yet, even here, up to half of the total lung capacity will remain unvisited by fresh air.

It is only through deep breathing that the lungs' complete capacity (C) is used – they completely fill and empty with each inhalation and exhalation. Once again, muscles move the ribs upward and outward, but this time the diaphragm also contracts and pulls downwards. Moreover, with deep breathing, the little-used lower lobe (D) of the right lung is utilised, which ensures that the maximum amount of stale air is expelled.

How important is it to expel this stale air?

Fresh air is unquestionably the most beneficial to you. Normally, though, when you exhale, some of the air in your lungs remains in either lungs or airways. This remaining air is called *anatomical dead space*. If we assume an average person inhales about 6000 cc (366 cu in) of air per minute (meaning there will be 6000 cc or 366 cu in of *stale* air to be exhaled), and has about 150 cc (9 cu in) of anatomical dead space, you can quickly see the effects the different types of breathing have.

BREATHING TYPE	VOL. AIR INHALED PER BREATH (cc)	BREATHS PER MIN. (6000 cc average vol. inhaled per min.)	VOL. DEAD SPACE PER MIN. (150 cc dead space X breaths per min.)	STALE AIR EXPELLED (average inhaled volume per min. – dead space per min.)
A1	150	40	6000	0
A2	250	24	3600	2400
B	500	12	1800	4200
C	1000	6	900	5100

An extremely shallow breather (A1), who has to breathe 40 times a minute, expels no stale air at all and would soon pass out. A typical shallow breather (A2) expels only a small proportion of the stale gases and is highly inefficient in the use of their lungs.

The ideal for everyday breathing is about twelve breaths a minute (B). *Instant calm* is encouraged by deep, slow breathing of even greater capacity (C). When deep breathing comes naturally – which it can with remarkable ease – you not only provide the maximum oxygen to your bloodstream, but you also expel the maximum volume of stale gases.

The bottom line? You will feel substantially more relaxed – almost immediately.

The art of breathing

There are three factors that play an influence on your breathing: habit, technique and posture.

Sometimes poor breathing is the product of many years' practice and cannot be easily corrected. Long-term bouts of shallow breathing cause a weakening of the diaphragm and abdominal muscles (breathing muscles), which limits their ability to function properly. Only by applying the correct technique can this be remedied.

One of the more obvious restrictions to correct breathing is your posture. Even the slightest slump of the shoulders can have an effect: it reduces the volume of your chest cavity which, in turn, causes you to breathe with your upper chest (shallow breathing) rather than your ribs and diaphragm.

Adjust your posture and amazing things become possible. Open up your chest cavity and greater quantities of air flood into your lower lungs. This, in turn, flushes more waste materials from them and eases muscular tensions around your stomach and rib areas. And as these tensions release, correct breathing becomes automatic.

However, even if you do alter your posture and concentrate on breathing deeply, you'll still be a long way from truly efficient deep breathing, because what we have discussed so far is merely the *principle* of correct breathing; the techniques that enable this are something else entirely.

Try this experiment. Take the deepest breath you are capable of. Suck in every bit of air your body can stand. Then some more. Now exhale.

Let's examine what you just did.

Invariably, your chest would have puffed out and your shoulders

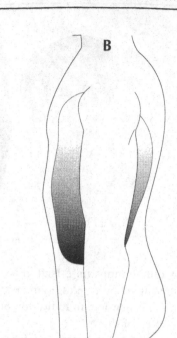

Figure 12

would have lifted. (Try it again in front of the mirror. This time, watch your chest and shoulders.) You would have heard a huge gushing intake of air. On exhalation, that air would have come rushing out almost explosively.

Do you think what you did was deep breathing? Do you think it would be humanly possible to squeeze even more air into those lungs?

If you examine Figures 12 and 13, you will note most people's idea of deep breathing (A) involves a substantial volume of air. But in doing this, the chest is puffed out, the upper portion of the lungs are inflated, and the whole procedure looks decidedly unnatural.

Examine (B), however, and you will see that the total lung capacity is significantly enlarged – without having to puff out the chest to any degree, and without raising the shoulders one centimetre. We call this Power Breathing.

Now hang on just one moment! Haven't we always been told,

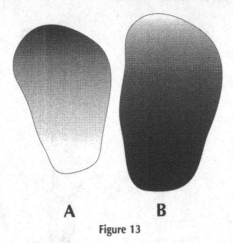

A   **B**

Figure 13

'Chest out, tummy in!'? Isn't this the guiding principle of proper breathing used by armies, gymnasiums and doctors' surgeries alike? Isn't chest expansion an indication of lung capacity?

Yes, to all of those.

But if you want to become proficient at Power Breathing, if you want to breathe completely and naturally, if you want to get more air into your lungs with less effort, if you want to understand why the 'breath of life' is called the breath of life, you will forget everything you've ever been told about this old 'chest out, tummy in' type of breathing.

The techniques which follow are incredibly simple. Once you know them, you will have a strength few others can equal.

And Power Breathing can become a vital and effortless part of your life.

12

POWER BREATHING

As any saxophonist, opera singer, meditator or martial artist will tell you, deep breathing or Power Breathing begins with your diaphragm. You already know that, you've heard it a thousand times. But, if you're like 99 per cent of the population, you will have only the vaguest idea what it means or how to achieve it.

The diaphragm is a sheet of muscle that divides the chest cavity and the abdominal cavity (see Figure 10). The chest cavity houses the lungs and is surrounded by a protective rib cage with the diaphragm forming its floor. In the act of deep breathing, contracting intercostal muscles move the ribs upward and outward while the diaphragm contracts and pulls downwards. This happens, to greater and lesser degrees, in all types of breathing.

When you inhale correctly, the diaphragm contracts downwards, allowing the lungs ample room to expand. When you exhale, the abdominal muscles push the diaphragm up against the lungs – this pushes the air out.

Power Breathing seeks more exertion from the diaphragm and rib cage than it does from the upper chest. In this way, the total lung capacity is significantly expanded, and breathing becomes easier and deeper. Why is that important? Because deep breathing causes your body to release endorphins, the tranquillising hormones.

All it takes is a few moments now and again to perfect the art.

The Plunger

I want you to visualise something. To do this you must forget all the diagrams and illustrations you have seen so far. Imagine your lungs as a single cylinder into which fresh air must be forced.

Now, as you take a breath of fresh air, imagine a plunger forcing that air down into the bottom of the cylinder. The top of the cylinder (your chest) does not expand in any way at all, but a flexible diaphragm at the bottom swells to accommodate the air.

That is how Power Breathing works.

Watch yourself in the mirror as you try it. First do it ensuring that your shoulders do not move. Once you have mastered that, try it without allowing your chest to puff out.

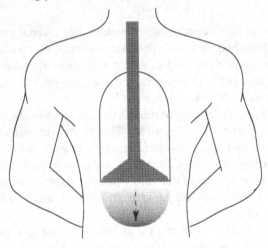

Figure 14

Now, hands on hips!

To get the feel of how your diaphragm expands when you are breathing correctly, place your hands on your hips (Figure 15), about level with your navel. Your thumbs will be resting in the hollow above each hip and your fingers will be resting on your stomach, stretching just below your navel.

Now, making sure your shoulders do not rise and your chest does not puff out, take a breath until you can feel your abdomen swell beneath your fingers and thumbs. Ensure your shoulders do not move.

As your diaphragm expands to accommodate your breath, you will feel your abdomen press out as well.

Now exhale slowly and evenly until you feel your abdomen fall.

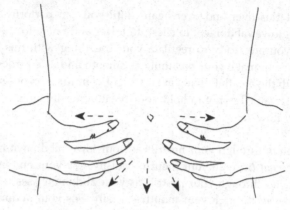

Figure 15

On your back!

This next exercise will be the one that makes Power Breathing as easy to perform as it is to understand. It requires you to lie flat on your back.

With your palms and outstretched fingers resting on your lower abdomen, distend your stomach muscles so that the entire lower stomach area protrudes (Figure 16a).

Once you have done this, suck in your stomach muscles as far as you can, which means that your chest will rise (Figure 16b).

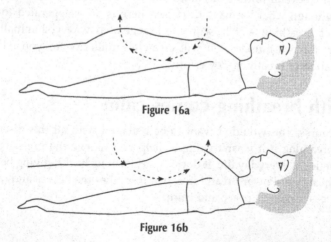

Figure 16a

Figure 16b

Repeat this over and over again until you can perform a rocking motion – lower abdomen, to chest, to lower abdomen, to chest . . .

Now you are ready to regulate your breathing with this muscular action. Try to make your breathing as smooth and as effortless as possible, with the breath flowing in and out of your lungs in one seemingly endless stream. Try not to hold your breath after inhaling.

Slowly now . . .

- Breathe *in* through your nostrils as your lower abdomen rises.
- Breathe *out* through your mouth – noisily – as your abdomen falls.
- Breathe *in* through your nostrils as your abdomen rises.
- Breathe *out* through your mouth – noisily – as your abdomen falls.
- Breathe *in* as your abdomen rises. Now 'force' the oxygen into the extremities of your body – your hands, feet and skull. Feel it coursing through your bloodstream to these parts.
- Breathe *out* – noisily – as your abdomen falls.

As you breathe out, *feel* the tension flood out of your body and into the floor. Feel it flow through your pores; feel it dissolve through the skin of your back at those places where it comes in contact with the floor. Feel your muscles relax as this tension flows out.

The pattern you are establishing here is the essence of Power Breathing. Continue that same muscular action when you are standing. Practise several times a day until you feel comfortable with it.

Although what we have discussed here is an exaggerated form of Power Breathing – at least in the exaggerated way you initially use your stomach muscles – it will create a familiarity for you with the sensation of breathing powerfully.

With breathing comes calm

Of course, you wouldn't want to be bothered with all this discussion on breathing if it wasn't going to help you relieve the pressures and anxieties of everyday life. It does! Apart from its health-giving benefits, the beauty of Power Breathing is that it soothes the nerves and quickly induces a state of peace and calm.

THE POWER BREATHING TECHNIQUE

- Remember the Conditions of Calm (see page 49).
- Take in a deep breath through your nostrils. Do this without exertion – neither raising your shoulders nor puffing out your chest.
- Hold it for a second. 'Force' the oxygen into the extremities of your body – your hands, feet and skull.
- Slowly breathe out, noisily, through your lips.
- Repeat a few times – smoothing out the inhalation and exhalation so there is one apparently seamless inflow and outflow of air.
- As you breathe out, feel the tension melting from your body into the floor. As the breathing becomes more automatic, concentrate on that tension passing from your body, through the soles of your feet (if you're standing), or through the skin of your back (if you're reclining) into the floor.

Now you know what people meant with the old saying, 'Take three deep breaths . . .'

IN CASE OF EMERGENCY
Exercise 1

This is based on the standard exercises in autogenic training, one of the common relaxation therapies taught by stress-control experts. The techniques will probably come as no surprise to you, but they are easy and they do work.

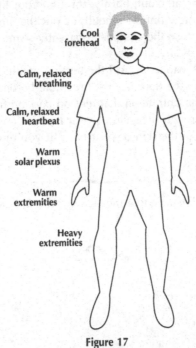

Cool
forehead

Calm, relaxed
breathing

Calm, relaxed
heartbeat

Warm
solar plexus

Warm
extremities

Heavy
extremities

Figure 17

STEP 1

Concentrate on the extremities of your body: your arms, legs, feet and hands. Feel them getting heavy. Repeat to yourself, over and over again, 'My left arm is heavy, my right arm is heavy, my left leg is heavy,' etc. Then: 'My arms and legs are heavy'.

STEP 2

Concentrate on the extremities of your body and feel them getting *warmer*. Repeat to yourself, over and over again, 'My arms and legs are warm'.

STEP 3

Now concentrate on your pulse rate (I prefer not to concentrate on heartbeats, but do so if you prefer). Feel it beating calmly. Repeat to yourself, over and over again, 'My pulse is calm and regular'.

STEP 4

Concentrate on your breathing. Listen to your breaths coming slowly and regularly. Repeat to yourself, over and over, 'My breathing is calm and regular'.

STEP 5

Concentrate on your solar plexus. Feel it getting warmer. Repeat to yourself, over and over again, 'My solar plexus is warm'.

STEP 6

Lastly concentrate on your forehead. Feel it getting cooler and cooler. Repeat to yourself, over and over, 'My forehead is cool'.

IN CASE OF EMERGENCY
Exercise 2

STEP 1
Mentally reassure yourself that good breathing is the
most effective way ever conceived to control feelings of stress
and anxiety.

STEP 2
Go somewhere quiet – even the bathroom will do at a pinch –
and take 30 seconds to gather your thoughts and to think about
what you're going to do.

STEP 3
Stand as erect as you can: feet flat, shoulders square, chin high.

STEP 4
Try to clear your mind – completely blank out all thoughts –
for a few moments.

STEP 5
If you feel comfortable doing so, assure yourself *out loud* that
you are feeling calm, you are feeling relaxed, you are a person
at peace.

STEP 6
Remembering not to raise your shoulders or to puff out your
chest while you do so, commence the Power Breathing
technique (see page 69).

13

CALM EXERCISES

Every book ever written on relaxation contains a series of muscle-relaxing exercises that can be performed while standing, sitting or reclining. They are as predictable as they are effective.

For reasons of tradition, I have included them. But if you consider them unimaginative or 'old hat', just pretend the next few paragraphs do not exist and go straight to The Answer from the East, page 76.

FIRST 'OLD FAITHFUL'

- Remember the Conditions of Calm (page 49).
- Either sitting, standing or reclining, really tense one set of muscles – such as the arms or legs.
- Now let them go limp! If you do this properly, the contrast between 'tense' and 'relaxed' should indicate what 'relaxed' really feels like. Dwell on that feeling.
- Now work on another set of muscles – such as the back, the stomach, the buttocks or the face.
- Now let them go limp! Dwell on the feeling of 'relaxed'. Savour it. Try to hang on to it.
- Repeat through all muscle groups.

SECOND 'OLD FAITHFUL'

- Remember the Conditions of Calm (page 49).
- Stand with your back against a wall. Feel the back of your head, your shoulders and your buttocks touching it.
- Breathing deeply, slowly raise your arms up to shoulder height as you breathe in.
- Wait 1 or 2 seconds.
- Slowly lower your hands and arms as you breathe out.
- Repeat this about 10 times, or longer if you feel it necessary.
- When complete, remain still and relaxed, breathing deeply, until you feel a sense of calm envelop you.

THIRD 'OLD FAITHFUL'

- While standing, breathe in and lift both shoulders slowly toward your ears for a couple of seconds.
- Breathing out, lower your shoulders to their normal position. Repeat this four or five times.
- Rotate your left shoulder (up, forward, down, back). Repeat with your right.
- Rotate both shoulders at once. Repeat four or five times.
- Reverse direction. Repeat four or five times.
- Relax your neck muscles. Let your head fall forward slowly until your chin rests on your chest. Return to the upright. Repeat four or five times.
- Slowly tilt your head towards your left shoulder. Return to the upright.
- Slowly tilt your head towards your right shoulder. Return to the upright.
- Repeat four or five times.
- Now, with your neck and shoulders relaxed, stand still and relaxed, breathing deeply.

The Answer from the East

No doubt you will have seen the peaceful, balletic movements of tai chi being practised. In China and Hong Kong, millions of ordinary citizens perform this ritual each morning.

Do they do it for the physical exercise? Possibly. More likely, however, they do it for the sense of peace and wellbeing that it encourages. Even to watch it is relaxing.

In its most basic form, tai chi is an intricate series of connected exercises which, combined, have the power to induce deep relaxation. They achieve this first of all by controlling the breathing, then by focusing the attention.

It is almost impossible to feel tense when performing their simple, graceful movements. You may find that the complete tai chi routine is difficult to learn and time-consuming to perform. Yet even elements of its routine, or the simple exercises that relate to it, can be powerfully relaxing in their own right. Following are three of them.

The most crucial aspect of each of these exercises is the beginning stance. Essentially, this is the same stance as is used in most martial arts – an unglamorous-looking pose that lowers your centre of gravity and 'fixes' you to the floor. In martial art applications, this makes you more ready to strike and to deflect, and more difficult to be thrown.

THE MARTIAL ARTS STANCE

- Feet should be positioned about a shoulder-width apart, with toes pointing straight ahead.
- Knees should be unlocked and slightly bent, perhaps even slightly bowed (even if they are not bowed, they should feel as if they are). You will feel a little muscular strain in the calves and backs of the thighs.
- Your elbows should be slightly bent and arms extended slightly out from the body – feel a little space under your armpits. Your hands should feel heavy and limp.
- Your back and neck should both be perfectly straight. Check this in a mirror if necessary. Your neck should be relaxed and you should be staring straight ahead.
- Concentrate your mass into your feet. You will feel your entire body weight sinking towards the floor. Feel it pressing down until it anchors you to the floor.

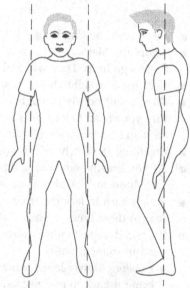

Figure 18

The Power Warm-up

This is a preparation exercise that can be employed alongside any of the techniques in this book. It is particularly appropriate as a preparation exercise for the two that follow it (the Windmill and the Power Stretch). It should be practised in conjunction with Power Breathing.

The secret of this exercise is to do it as slowly as you possibly can; the slower you do it, the more beneficial it is.

THE POWER WARM-UP

- Remember the Conditions of Calm.
- Adopt the Martial Arts Stance. Let your arms, wrists and fingers go limp. They will feel heavy and relaxed.
- Eyes fixed straight ahead, slowly breathe in.
- Breathe out noisily through your lips and, as you do, slowly turn your head to look over your *right* shoulder. Keep your back and neck in a straight line; and do not move shoulders.
- Breathing in, slowly return your head to the front.
- As you breathe out noisily through your lips, slowly turn your head to look over your *left* shoulder.
- Slowly turn to face the front again.
- Repeat three times in each direction.
- If desired, repeat entire exercise, substituting right-to-left head movement with:
  - *Exhaling*, slowly lower your head to your chest; *inhaling*, bring it back to upright; slowly lean it back so you are looking to the ceiling; slowly bring it back to upright.
  - *Exhaling*, slowly lean your head to the left; *inhaling*, bring it back to upright; slowly lean it to the right; bring it back.

The Power Stretch

This simple exercise is profoundly calming. It works almost immediately and requires no strain or athletic prowess to succeed. *Endeavour to do it as slowly and as gracefully as you can manage.*

While at first it may appear complex, the Power Stretch is really quite simple and straightforward. After you've performed it a couple of times, the movements will flow quite intuitively.

Fundamentally, there are three coordinated actions (each one very simple) contained within the one exercise.

1 Control of breathing.
2 The raising of the hands and arms.
3 The stretching of the body from toes to finger tips.

Once again, coordination of the three becomes second nature after you have performed this a couple of times.

For maximum efficacy, you may choose to precede the Power Stretch with the Power Warm-up exercise.

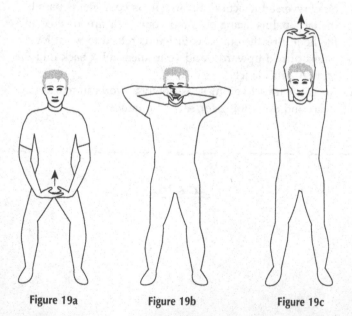

Figure 19a   Figure 19b   Figure 19c

THE POWER STRETCH

- Remember the Conditions of Calm.
- Adopt the Martial Arts Stance. Let your arms, wrists and fingers go limp. They will feel heavy and relaxed.
- Loosely entwine your fingers. Turn your palms so that they face upwards.
- (i) Slowly breathe in. (ii) Raise cupped hands towards the mouth – as if drawing water from a well. (iii) Begin to straighten legs so your body is straight.
- (i) Slowly begin to breathe out. (ii) Turn cupped hands so the palms face out. (iii) Begin to stretch out your body. (Figure 19b.)
- (i) Slowly exhale all air. (ii) Arms reach upwards and palms now face the ceiling. (iii) Body is stretched out, you are standing on your toes. (Figure 19c.)
- Now reverse the action. Breathe in as your hands pass by the face, palms facing out, and your heels are lowered to the floor. Breathe out as your hands return to waist level, palms turned upwards, and your knees relax back into the Martial Arts Stance.
- Repeat at least five times, as slowly as you can manage.
- Relax and do nothing for several minutes.

The Windmill

Have you ever seen a Dutch windmill turning? Graceful, relaxed, effortless. Imagine just such a scene – but in *slow motion*! This, as you might have guessed, is the key to the Windmill.

Nothing could be easier than this particular exercise. Anyone can do it – I know, because I mastered it myself after only five minutes – it requires no athletic skills, and it works beautifully every time.

Essentially, there is nothing more to the Windmill than this: the arms sweep upwards in one big, circular movement as you rise up onto your toes; then the arms return to complete the circle at about waist level while your knees relax back into the Martial Arts Stance. You breathe in as your arms (and your lungs) are at their widest (that is, closest to horizontal), and breathe out as they cross above your head or at your waist.

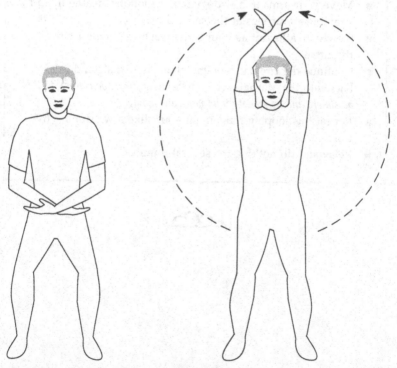

Figure 20

Once again, endeavour to do this *as slowly and as gracefully as you can manage.*

For maximum efficacy, you may choose to precede the Windmill with the Power Warm-up exercise.

THE WINDMILL

- Remember the Conditions of Calm.
- Adopt the Martial Arts Stance. Let your arms, wrists and fingers go limp. They will feel heavy and relaxed. Cross your wrists at about waist level, palms facing upwards.
- Move your arms in a wide, circular motion. Breathe in and straighten your legs at the same time.
- Slowly breathe out as your arms reach the highest part of the circle.
- Continue the circular movement as you exhale and relax back into the Martial Arts Stance. *Remember, you must do this as slowly and as smoothly as you can manage.*
- Repeat this looping movement – just like a windmill – five times.
- Relax and do nothing for several minutes.

14

CALM
SUGGESTION

The subconscious is a powerful force.

Unlike the conscious mind, however, the subconscious has no ability to discriminate: under the right conditions, any suggestion that is presented to it will be taken on board and acted upon.

This fundamental understanding is what makes a great salesperson great, is what causes normally healthy people to fall ill, is what causes terminally ill people to effect complete recovery, is what causes martial art champions to triumph over opposition, and is what allows professional golfers to win.

This understanding is also the basis of hypnosis.

Most stress-related problems are the result of activities of the subconscious. If you are to overcome such problems – if you are to become calm and relaxed at all times – you need to harness your subconscious. Push the right 'buttons', and it will work more powerfully for the positive than it will for the negative.

Suggestion can be a real pain

Why is it that if you talk of your work being a real pain in the neck you begin to develop tense neck muscles whenever you're there? Why is it that when someone details a serious ailment affecting them, *you* begin to feel the symptoms? Why is it that when you talk of your father-in-law being a real headache, you develop a migraine whenever he's around? Why is it that a discussion on itching causes you to scratch? Why is it that failures spend so much time talking about failure?

Coincidence? Not at all. This phenomenon is known as 'applied suggestion'. It can emanate from someone else (such as a complainer, or a hypnotist) or from yourself; either way, once that suggestion is accepted by the subconscious, the subconscious sets about transforming it into reality.

Thus, if you tell yourself you're feeling lousy (especially if you tell yourself sufficient times, or if you tell yourself persuasively enough) then there can be nothing surer than you're going to feel lousy. Similarly, if you tell yourself you're never going to make that putt, then there is nothing surer than you're never going to make that putt. It's as simple as that.

Examine your own life and you will see example after example after example.

How can you make this discovery work for you? Easy. If you keep on telling yourself *positive* things, *calming* things, then you will achieve them. If you are persistent, this *will* work; there is nothing surer. But don't celebrate yet: it gets even better!

> The subconscious must be seduced into responding the way you want it to. To be effective, therefore, the ideas you plant in it must appeal to the imagination rather than the intellect.

More powerful still is *visual* suggestion. If you can *see* these positive things, these calming things, and especially if you can 'see' yourself participating in them, then you are certainly well down the track towards achieving them.

What follows will show you how, through simple use of language and mental pictures, you can make yourself feel better.

Instantly.

Imagination versus Willpower

Many believe that by applying sufficient willpower, they can achieve whatever they set their minds to. They believe sheer weight of will overcomes any subconscious urge or compulsion.

Nothing could be further from the truth.

As far as the subconscious is concerned, imagination wins out over will every time. Every time. Imagination usually wins out over logic and common sense as well.

You know that your chances of being attacked by a great white shark are around one in a billion. You also know that you stand a much greater chance of being struck by lightning, or run over by a bus. Why, then, does your heart-rate soar as your legs dangle beneath the surfboard, yet hardly alters when you're caught in an electrical storm or when you're crossing a busy road?

Imagination.

Worse, the imagination escalates in multiple proportions to the exertion of your will. Continuing the shark analogy: the more you try to use willpower *not* to think about great white sharks, the more you'll fear them as your legs dangle beneath the surfboard.

The will is a tool of your conscious mind; for it to function effectively, it must operate in accord with what exists in your *subconscious mind.

On the other hand, the subconscious is all dreams, emotions, fuzzy things, abstract ideas, concepts, pictures, ideals. For it to accept one of your logical, hard-edged, black and white, practical demands – that is, a command from your will – it has to be *seduced* into responding the way you want it to.

If you want to influence the way you think and feel, therefore, the suggestions you take on board must appeal to the *imagination* rather than the intellect.

If you were asked to walk the length of a plank that was lying on the floor, you'd do it with the greatest of ease.

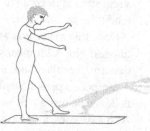

Suspend that plank between two tall buildings, however, and the task becomes immense.
Why?
Because of your imagination.

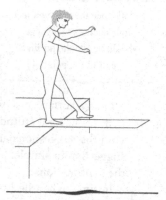

Your choice of suggestions

Remember how applied suggestion works? Once a suggestion is accepted by the subconscious, it is transformed into reality. *Once it is accepted by the subconscious.*

To ensure that a suggestion is acceptable to the subconscious, it should be in harmony – or at least not be in conflict – with suggestions that are already present.

In other words, it's no good telling yourself you're 'a six-foot superman' if your subconscious knows you are five feet one and skinny. It may be easier to convince yourself that you're 'strong and walk tall'. The difference is nothing more than your choice of words – the first suggestion is in conflict with what already exists in your subconscious, while the second is more acceptable.

Does this mean you are condemned to perpetuate any negative self-images? No. All it means is that you should choose positive suggestions that are *generally* in accord with what you accept about yourself.

Suppose a person wanted to feel like a success, a winner, yet genuinely believed he was a real loser who had continually been dealt badly by fate. As his subconscious has undoubtedly been conditioned to think that way, it would be pointless applying the suggestion, 'I am recognised as the most popular man in the world', or 'I am recognised as the most successful man in the world', because these are in discord with the suggestions already in his subconscious. He could, however, use a suggestion along the lines of: 'More and more, I am discovering that my positive attitude attracts good fortune and interesting people'. And, more importantly, it would work for him!

> To influence the way you feel, your choice of language should be simple, positive and to the point.

Notice how the words are couched in the present ('I am discovering') as opposed to the future ('I am going to discover').

On the surface, a suggestion such as this may appear to be in conflict with his general attitude towards himself. But it is not a *direct* conflict with the suggestions already there. And, because he has couched the suggestion in simple, positive terms, it appears far more acceptable to the subconscious.

In time, when he *has* begun to change the attitudes resident in his subconscious, maybe he could get away with the suggestion, 'I am recognised as the most popular man in the world', and have it work for him. Because such is the power of suggestion.

Your choice of words

As any hypnotist will tell you, the words you use (or the words you listen to and believe) have a profound effect on the way you feel. Particularly when those words are framed in the present.

Try to imagine how you'd feel if a stranger came up to you and said: 'You're looking wonderful.' You'd feel lighter and happier from that moment on.

What if that stranger had said: 'You looked wonderful last week'? Or 'If you buy that shirt you'll look wonderful'? Not the same, is it?

That's why hypnotic language is always framed in the present: 'You are feeling sleepy. Your eyelids are heavy, you are finding it difficult to keep them apart.'

> If you want to influence your subconscious, repeat, repeat, repeat.

Even more importantly, your choice of language should be simple, positive and to the point. When trying to influence your subconscious, there is no room for sub-clauses and qualifications, just simple, straightforward, positive suggestions. 'I am enjoying my life more and more. Every moment of it becomes more and more fulfilling.' (I feel better just for having written that.)

Time and time again

You've watched how hypnotists work on television: they make the same suggestion over and over again. Perhaps they rephrase it in different ways, but they repeat and repeat.

Repetition forces a suggestion into the subconscious. Just as it takes many months or years of negative suggestions to turn someone into a failure, or an accident-prone or ill person, it takes many repetitions of *positive* suggestions to counter this.

More importantly, repetition tends to drive away unnecessary conscious thoughts. It simply leaves no room for them to exist. This enables you to concentrate in ways sheer willpower will never enable you to do. When you can concentrate like this – that is, not through willpower, but through the *absence* of conscious thought – your subconscious will be at its most receptive.

And if you want to influence your subconscious, repeat, repeat, repeat.

Calm Affirmation

Affirmation is a technique that is well known to the religious, to hypnotists, hypnotherapists, psychotherapists, promoters of self-help courses and, most of all, producers of self-help audio tapes. It is the process of auto-suggestion or, as some like to call it, self-instruction.

Affirmations are a specially conceived set of words that, by being repeated over and over to yourself, influence the subconscious and become self-fulfilling. Through carefully chosen words or sentiments, you project the results you desire to take place.

Affirmation is an enormously powerful technique for long-term change. But it also has profound powers for immediate change.

For immediate change

Like many of the techniques in this book, my suggestion for using affirmations to effect an immediate change in your mood may seem over-simplified. Indeed, for many readers, acceptance of this may also require a leap of faith.

Be assured, though, that if you embrace this technique enthusiastically, it will work for you.

The key is to be creative with the wording of your affirmation. For example, if the cause of your anxiety is fear of failing at something or other, then you must choose words that are the antithesis of 'fear' for your affirmation. Recite the following words to yourself – emphatically – and feel the difference they make to the way you feel.

I feel total confidence in my skills and abilities.

I know that I can achieve anything I set my mind to.

I radiate this confidence to all around me.

Note the use of simple, active, positive words. Note the use of the present tense. Note the use of emotive words ('feel', 'radiate') which appeal to the imagination rather than the intellect.

As another example: if you are angry over some minor (in the universal scale of things) transgression of a friend or lover, you can transform that anger into something far more positive.

I am charged with the most powerful feelings of love and camaraderie for those who are near to me. I radiate those feelings and they are reciprocated.

As a third example, here is an affirmation for someone suffering non-specific feelings of tension and anxiety.

More and more, I am relaxing into a state of great peace and calm. I am feeling content, tranquil and at ease with the world. I radiate this peace and calm to all I come in contact with.

Keep repeating these words to yourself – as loudly as the environment you are in will allow – until they fill your consciousness. Repeat, repeat, repeat. Do it for at least five minutes. If your mind wanders, just keep reciting the words when you are aware of it, without bothering to take in their meaning.

As a sure way of emphasising the positive values of your words, try substituting the following for their more negative counterparts.

FOR THIS *NEGATIVE* . . .	SUBSTITUTE THIS *POSITIVE*
Fear	Confidence
Failure	Success
Illness	Health
Anger	Love
Chaos	Calm
Panic	Peace
Miserable	Happy
Empty	Fulfilled
Can't	Can
Maybe	Possible
Loss	Win
Depressed	Uplifted
Bored	Stimulated

IMMEDIATE AFFIRMATION TECHNIQUE

- Remember the Conditions of Calm.
- Commence slow Power Breathing. Continue for at least 1 minute.
- Choose positive words/phrases that:
  - reflect how you would ideally like to be;
  - are simple, active, positive and to the point;
  - are in the *present*;
  - appeal to the imagination, rather than the intellect.
- Keep repeating these words to yourself. Repeat, repeat, repeat.

Long-term affirmations

There is a variety of other ways of using affirmations which, even though they may take longer to achieve maximum results, have the capacity to effect more dramatic and sustainable changes than the ones already outlined.

The simplest of these ways is the Ten Ten technique.

Briefly, the formula for this technique is to take a set of words – a positive, active set of words that reflect the way you'd like to be or to feel – then to repeat those words out aloud ten times, and to repeat this exercise ten times throughout the day.

Ten times. Ten times a day.

THE TEN TEN TECHNIQUE

- Remember the Conditions of Calm.
- Commence slow Power Breathing. Continue for at least 1 minute.
- Choose positive words or phrases that reflect how you would ideally like to be. Choose words that are simple, active, positive and to the point. And in the present tense. Use words that appeal to the imagination, not the intellect.
- Repeat these words to yourself 10 times.
- Repeat this exercise 10 times throughout the day.

15

CALM VISUALISATION

Visualisation is the most powerful technique you can employ for influencing the subconscious and for effecting change – because of its unsurpassed appeal to the imagination (which is, after all, the picture-forming faculty of the mind).

You've heard the cliché, 'a picture is worth a thousand words'. Nowhere is this more true than in influencing the subconscious. The road accident you witness is much harder to forget than the one that is described to you; a poor haircut is much more shocking in the reflection of a shop window than it is in a description over the telephone; the glimpse of a beautiful woman in the flesh is infinitely more memorable than a florid description of her in the newspaper columns.

It follows, therefore, that if you could feed the subconscious with positive *images*, as opposed to positive suggestions, then the level of influence would be significantly greater.

The power of the picture

Through carefully chosen mental pictures or visual concepts, you can project onto your subconscious the outcomes you desire. Applied correctly and creatively, these images can transform your life.

However, unlike reciting affirmations, visualisations require a certain level of imaginative skill. The question many people ask is, 'Do I have this skill?'

As you know, we all have five senses: auditory (hearing), visual (seeing), kinaesthetic (touch), taste and smell. In most people, there is one dominant sense, usually either auditory, visual or kinaesthetic. For those whose dominant sense is visual, the ability to visualise comes easily and naturally. In fact, they respond most strongly to images, and process most of life's information in a visual way.

Sometimes, however, those whose dominant sense is auditory or kin-aesthetic believe they cannot visualise at all. They are wrong, of course, everyone can visualise. But because visualisation relates more to the subconscious and can be directed only to a certain degree by the conscious mind, it may seem somewhat difficult to certain individuals.

> Because visualisation relates to imagination (and the subconscious), it may appear difficult for some individuals. Even though it is not difficult, and is within all our capabilities and everyday experiences, it may still seem unattainable. In such cases, simply pretend that you can visualise. By pretending, you trick your subconscious into believing – the effect will be exactly the same.

I remember at one particular seminar I was attending, a woman claimed to be incapable of visualising anything. 'I just can't visualise,' she moaned. 'I have no imagination.'

We told her not to even try, just to *pretend* she could visualise. Just to take her time and pretend she could do it. That is exactly what she did – she pretended. And guess what? Her visualisations were perfect. By pretending, she fooled her subconscious into believing, and everything went smoothly from that moment on.

You can use visualisation as easily as that. If you doubt your ability to visualise, simply pretend that you can. It will work just as effectively.

Following are several visualisation techniques. Try them out, work on them – you'll find they can be singularly powerful.

Big Screen Visualisation

This has been designed for the modern-day visualiser. It employs 'technology' – or the visual tools of technology – with which we are all familiar and comfortable. Instead of trying to imagine or visualise in some poorly defined area of your mind, you imagine it happening up there on a big screen.

This is how it works. (Do all of what follows with closed eyes.) First, choose an image that best sums up the way you would like to feel.

If you're feeling overworked and highly stressed, the image you

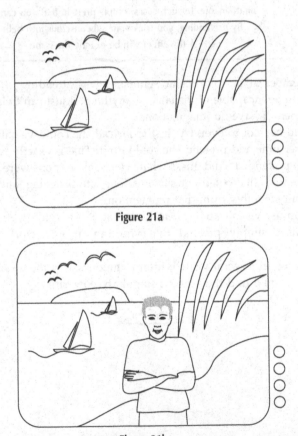

Figure 21a

Figure 21b

choose might be one of yourself at the peak of a beautiful, snowcapped mountain. Or on an idyllic South Pacific island.

The next step is to imagine this image being played on a big screen television set. Or, if you're the showy type, on a large cinema screen.

With eyes closed, 'look' at the image on that screen: the long stretches of tropical beach, the vast expanses of alpine slopes. And when you can see it clearly, *step inside the image.*

See yourself up there, standing on the sun-bleached sands of that tropical island. Note what you're wearing, the relaxed way you're standing, the way the breeze blows your hair, the calm, semi-smile on your face.

Now 'see' the scene as you would see it if you were really there.

Next 'hear' the sounds of that environment as if you were really there. The waves lapping at the shore. The seagulls. The breeze in the trees.

Then 'feel' what it is like to be there. The warmth of the sun on your body. The cool breeze on your face. The way your feet sink into the soft sand as you walk.

And, when you feel that you are really experiencing being there, it's time for the technological bit.

Reach for the volume and picture 'controls' of your imaginary big screen set.

Turn both of them up. More, more.

The picture becomes brighter and brighter. The sounds grow louder. And, as a result, the physical manifestations also become more pronounced, the feelings more intense.

Within seconds, you're feeling calm and relaxed – as if you really were on that wonderful island of your imagination.

THE BIG SCREEN VISUALISATION

- Remember the Conditions of Calm.
- Commence slow Power Breathing. Continue for at least 1 minute.
- Close your eyes.
- Think of the most relaxed environment you can imagine. 'See' that image on a big screen set inside your mind. Examine it in detail.
- Now step inside that image. See yourself up there, totally involved in it. Note how you react to the environment or the elements.
- Then 'see' all the scenery surrounding you.
- 'Hear' all the sounds about you.
- 'Feel' the physical aspects of the place you're in.
- When that image is firmly implanted in your mind, *turn up* the picture and the sound.
- Relax, keeping that sense of calm with you. (If necessary, repeat the exercise.)

The Superimposition Technique

Here's another visualisation technique designed for the visually oriented. Although some people may find it difficult to do, I've included it here because it is a powerful technique used by some psychotherapists.

The Superimposition Technique consists of two parts: you as you are feeling at that moment (tense and stressed), and you as you would *like* to feel (relaxed and worry free).

As in the previous technique, you visualise both of these people up on your imaginary big screen (Figure 22a).

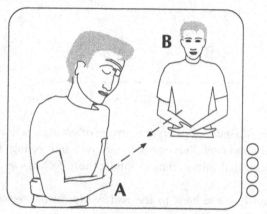

Figure 22a

Start with a picture of yourself as you are at that moment (A); that should not be hard to do. Keep the image to the lower left-hand side of your screen.

Once you are comfortable with that image, conjure up a picture of yourself as you would like to be (B) – relaxed and worry free. You may need to recall some time in the past when you felt like that. If you like, relive that experience, trying to recall what you saw, what you heard, what you felt at that time.

Keep this image – complete with the sounds and feelings – to the upper right of your screen. Please remember that it is important that your ideal is on the upper right.

Now slowly bring the two images together.

Keep bringing them together until you have *superimposed* the ideal picture of yourself over the other (Figure 22b).

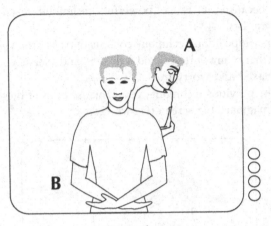

Figure 22b

Once the relaxed and worry free image of yourself is dominant, hold it there for a moment. Remember the sounds and feelings that go with it. Keep with that image, those sounds, those feelings as long as you can.

Then slowly come back to the real world, bringing with you that experience of being relaxed and worry free.

And you will be relaxed and worry free. It's as easy as that.

THE SUPERIMPOSITION TECHNIQUE

- Remember the Conditions of Calm.
- Commence slow Power Breathing.
- Close your eyes and formulate a picture of yourself *as you are now* on your mental 'big screen'.
- Now formulate a picture of *yourself feeling relaxed and worry free.* Keep this picture to the upper right. 'See' yourself up there, totally involved in it. Note the detail: the sounds, what you're doing, what you're feeling.
- Then slowly bring the two images together until the relaxed one totally covers the present one.
- Stay with that image for as long as you can.
- When your relaxed image blocks out the worried one, turn up the brightness and volume on your big screen. See the pictures more clearly. Hear the sounds more loudly.
- Relax, bringing that experience of being relaxed and worry free back with you.

Stepping Into Time

Here is yet another visualisation technique – but this one is even more refined than those already covered.

This technique is much simpler to perform than it may at first appear. Persevere; it will be well worth the effort.

Stepping Into Time is a mixture of the physical (distance and movement) with imagination (visualisation). This confusion of reality and imagination is a highly effective way of overcoming the barriers your conscious mind erects to keep you feeling stressed. By satisfying your left brain (distance, movement) and right brain (creating mental pictures) at the same time,

As with the other techniques in this book, do not be fooled into mistaking simplicity for lack of effectiveness; visualisations are powerful mood- and attitude-changing techniques, often employed for more profound psychological treatments than stress control.

you charm the subconscious into allowing you to feel relaxed and worry free, or to feel happy and self-confident – whatever you choose.

Stepping Into Time requires you to project an ideal of yourself – how you'd like to be, how you'd like to feel – some way into the future. How far into the future does not matter at all: it could be two hours, four months, ten years even.

Do all of what follows while you're standing. Choose a room where there is at least 2–3 metres (6–10 feet) space in front of you.

Where you are standing is 'the present'.

Close your eyes and imagine the future stretching out before you (Figure 23a). Don't worry about the distance, just think about the future. Imagine all this on your 'big screen'.

Some physical distance away – that is, way off in the future – you can see, or imagine, yourself as you would like to be (Figure 23b). You'll be relaxed, contented and worry free, of course. Imagine what it feels like to be like that: the sounds you'll hear, the things you'll feel, the activity you might be participating in. If necessary, refer back to some experience in your past so that you can conjure a sufficient level of realism.

When you can 'see', 'hear' and 'feel' what it will be like on that future occasion, become aware of yourself in the present. Formulate a picture

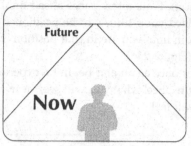

Figure 23a

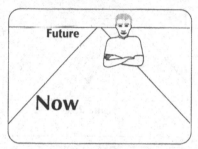

Figure 23b

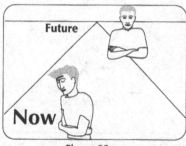

Figure 23c

of yourself as you are right now – probably at the lower left of your screen – all stressed and anxious (Figure 23c).

Open your eyes.

Note the approximate place in that room where your mental picture of the future was positioned.

Now step away to the left, away from your 'present'. Move out at least a metre (3 feet). Walk a few paces ahead until you are level with where you imagined your 'future' to be positioned.

Now step back in until you are in that position where you imagined the future to be (Figure 23d).

Close your eyes once again and begin to 'experience' what you will be like in the future. 'See' what you will see; 'hear' what you will hear; 'feel' what you will feel.

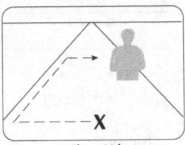

Figure 23d

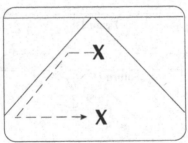

Figure 23e

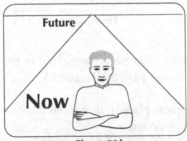

Figure 23f

When you can experience this fully, step out to the side again, and retrace your steps to the 'present' – bringing that experience of the future back with you (Figure 23e). Hold that feeling with you as you re-integrate it with the present (Figure 23f).

This is a major attitude-changing technique that has the potential to produce permanent change.

STEPPING INTO TIME

- Choose a place with 2–3 metres (6–10 feet) clear space in front of you.
- Close your eyes. Commence slow Power Breathing. Continue for at least 1 minute.
- On your big screen, 'see' the future stretch out in front of you.
- 'See' yourself as you would like to be – relaxed, contented and worry free – at some indeterminate time in the future. 'See' yourself there, totally involved in the experience. Note the details of it: the sounds, what you are doing, what you are feeling.
- Now become aware of yourself right now – in the 'present'.
- Physically take a step to the left. Walk forward until you become level with the position you imagined your future image to be. Step into that position.
- 'Experience' what it is like to be in that future position. Note all that surrounds you, the sounds, the feelings. Note how calm and relaxed you are.
- Step to the side again, and retrace your steps to the 'present'. Bring that relaxed, worry free experience back with you.
- Hold that feeling as you re-integrate it with the present.

Framing

Some public-speaking courses advocate the following technique for nervous speakers: imagine your audience sitting stark naked in front of you, or imagine your audience not as a group of human beings but as a group of monkeys.

Personally, I'd feel pretty strange standing up there fully clothed in

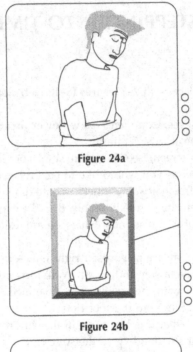

Figure 24a

Figure 24b

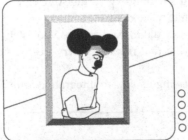

Figure 24c

front of a naked audience, or speaking to a roomful of gorillas. But I'm assured that the technique works for many public speakers.

Why?

Because the public speaker *reframed* his/her fears or anxieties (in this case, an audience) into one that was not only less threatening, but possibly even amusing.

As basic as that technique may appear, it is not far removed from another used for treating phobias and irrational fears. This also uses the 'framing' metaphor with great effectiveness. It can be modified to treat everyday problems like tension and stress.

To begin with, framing requires you to be able to visualise your fear. Or to visualise yourself (Figure 24a) in whatever state is bothering you – stress, anxiety, tension.

Allow that image to take form on your big screen. Note the surrounding *visual* details: the images that accompany it, the environment you are situated in.

When that picture is well formulated, mentally put it inside a cute little wooden frame. See it as a harmless, nicely framed little picture (Figure 24b).

Now it is time to have some fun.

After your fear or anxiety is neatly contained in that little frame, experiment with redefining it. Remember, the object of this is to make your worries look as trivial and as harmless as possible.

If it's your angry, cigar-smoking boss that distresses you, try to picture him with Shirley Temple curls and wearing a floral nightdress. If your picture is of yourself in a state of extreme anxiety add a funny nose and a clown costume, or Mickey Mouse ears, or whatever it takes to remove the serious edge from your feelings (Figure 24c).

Then turn up the 'brightness control' on your big screen.

Later, should any re-occurrence of your fear or anxiety appear, simply conjure up your redefined image of it, and be amazed at how quickly it ceases to have any negative effect on you.

THE FRAMING TECHNIQUE

- Remember the Conditions of Calm. Sit in a comfortable chair. Remove your shoes.
- Begin Power Breathing.
- On your big screen conjure up an image of yourself under stress. Or an image of your fear. Concentrate on the *visual* details surrounding it.
- Place that image in a cute little wooden frame. Note the details of the entire picture – you or your fear, plus the cute little wooden frame.
- Have some fun with the image in the frame. Make it amusing and harmless. Maybe fit Mickey Mouse ears to it.
- When you have redefined the image, turn up the 'brightness control' on your big screen.
- If your fear or anxiety resurfaces, simply recall that trivialised image from the frame.

Calming Self-hypnosis

You know how hypnosis is meant to work. In many ways, it is just as you've seen it so many times on television variety shows. You've probably read about self-hypnosis, too, and more than likely have imagined it as something equally as mysterious and magical.

This is not necessarily so.

The essential difference between the two is who calls the shots. In one instance, you open your subconscious to the guidance of another person – the hypnotist; in the second, you conduct the entire business yourself. In both instances, though, *you* are responsible for all that takes place.

Earlier in this chapter you learned about applied suggestion and how, through affirmation and visualisation, it can influence your subconscious. The difference between making those suggestions in a waking state or in a hypnotic state is one of degree.

So, how do you perform self-hypnosis?

One way is to visit a hypnotist and get him or her to give you a post-hypnotic suggestion that allows you to enter self-hypnosis when and as you decide. Most people, however, will choose to use the simple technique that follows.

The first and most important consideration about calming self-hypnosis is to realise how 'normal' it really is. Contrary to what television shows would have you believe, it has nothing to do with dangling watches or swirling spirals: it is simply a process of 'filling up the senses' until you attain a highly focused state.

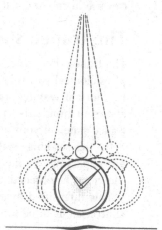

The secret of self-hypnosis

All hypnosis consists of two parts: (a) inducing a trance, and (b) presenting a suggestion that your subconscious will turn into a reality.

Even though the word 'trance' by itself is usually enough to conjure up all sorts of dark and mysterious images, it is a natural, everyday event that each and every one of us has experienced.

Yes, even you.

Have you ever been on train ride, with nothing to do but look out the window and listen to the clickety-clack of the wheels? Do you recall on that occasion how you 'stared into space', 'daydreaming', 'not really thinking about anything'? That was a trance. Very likely it was every bit as deep and meaningful – for however brief a period – as any hypnotic trance.

Okay, so you hate trains. Have you even been given a massage, a facial, or even a haircut and found yourself 'daydreaming', possibly even 'nodding off'?

That's right, a trance.

You did not 'fall into a deep sleep', nor did you lose control. It may have been for only a few minutes, it may have been only a few seconds, but it was a trance. Exactly the same sort of trance that Mandrake the Magician uses up there on stage. Exactly the same sort of trance you can use in calming self-hypnosis.

The trance state

The trance state differs from the normal waking state in a number of physiological ways. The most significant of these is your attention. In the normal waking state, you can take in many things, you can be aware of hundreds of different stimuli all at the same time; in the trance state, all your attention is focused on one area.

In the waking state, your awareness is broad, flat and all-encompassing; in the trance state, your awareness is focused and, therefore, heightened and more intense.

This intensified awareness in the trance state is what causes your subconscious to be so receptive to suggestion.

Inducing a trance

There are a thousand ways to bring about the trance state, but the one I favour has a 'proof' stage incorporated into it.

Essentially, it consists of filling up the senses with your own observations, then narrowing those observations down one by one until your attention is focused. This is the trance state.

Find yourself a comfortable place to sit in a dimly lit room. Ensure you will not be interrupted. Take off your shoes, wear loose clothes, and make sure you're warm.

Before you begin anything, tell yourself several times that the moment you reach the trance state, your right hand will begin to rise. Slowly, surely, and of its own accord. This will be a signal from your subconscious that you have reached the trance state. (There is no mystery about how this works: it's just like the 'mental alarm clock' we are all familiar with – you tell yourself several times before dozing off that you're going to wake at five a.m., and sure enough you'll wake at five a.m.)

Leave your hands apart, resting comfortably on your lap.

Find one bright thing in the room that you can focus on. Maybe it's the red stand-by light on your television set. Maybe it's a reflection on a brass door handle or a highlight on a white vase. Fix your attention on that bright spot. (The objective is to continue focusing on that spot throughout the exercise.)

Now, *using only your peripheral vision*, without letting your eyes move from that visual highlight you have chosen, **note six different things you can see** in that room. 'I can see the light switch. I can see the corner of the sofa. I can see the standard lamp. I can see the photograph of Grandma. I can see the Persian carpet. I can see my hands on my knees.'

Next, without allowing your eyes to stray from that visual highlight, **note six different sounds you can hear**. 'I can hear the clock ticking. I can hear the tap dripping in the bathroom. I can hear the sound of my own breathing. I can hear the hum of the air-conditioner. I can hear a motorcycle passing. I can hear crickets in the garden.'

Once again, without allowing your eyes to stray from that visual highlight, **note six different things you can feel**. 'I can feel the carpet under my feet. I can feel the chair against my legs. I can feel my belt sticking into my hip. I can feel my back resting against the chair. I can feel a draught coming from the window. I can feel my elbows resting against my body.'

The next time around, note only five of those things you can see. And hear. And feel. (All the while make sure to keep focusing on that highlight.)

Then note only four things.

And three.

And two.

And one.

Then you will probably notice that your hand has drifted upwards of its own accord. You will probably get such a surprise that you will jar yourself out of the trance state at that instant. (This last part of the process, the automatically rising hand, is nothing more than a once-only trick to demonstrate how your subconscious will communicate with you. Place too much importance on it and you may inhibit the process. If so, it is not important.)

Presenting the suggestion

Remember the segment on affirmations? All of those affirmations you created then are the autosuggestions you can use in calming self-hypnosis.

Say, for example, that the following encompassed everything that you would like to achieve through your calming self-hypnosis.

More and more, I am relaxing into a state of great peace and calm. I am feeling content, tranquil and at ease with the world. I radiate this peace and calm to all I come in contact with.

The object of calming self-hypnosis is to feed those words to your subconscious after you have reached the trance state. There are two easy ways of doing this.

The first is simply to have repeated them to yourself so many times that you know them by heart. Then, at the outset of your calming self-hypnosis session, instead of telling yourself that your right hand is going to rise, tell yourself that you are going to recite your affirmation once you have reached the trance state. Your subconscious will take care of the rest.

Alternatively, record your affirmation on a tape recorder and, at the outset of your calming self-hypnosis session, instruct yourself to turn on your message once you have reached the trance state.

CALMING SELF-HYPNOSIS

- Remember the Conditions of Calm. Sit in a comfortable chair. Remove your shoes. Rest your hands apart, comfortably on your lap.
- Tell yourself that you're going to recite your affirmations (autosuggestions) once you enter the trance state. Alternatively, tell yourself that you're going to play a pre-recorded tape.
- Concentrate on one visual bright spot in the room – continue to focus on that spot throughout.
- Note six different things you can *see* in that room. Using only your peripheral vision, note them one by one.
- Note six different things you can *hear*. Without taking your eyes from that bright spot, note them one by one.
- Note six different things you can *feel*.
- Then note *five* different things you can see. And hear. And feel.
- Note four. And three. And two. And one.
- Recite affirmations to yourself. Alternatively, play the pre-recorded tape.

Let's Pretend

WORRIER: 'I find it impossible to relax. I've tried every technique, but I still find it impossible to relax.'

THERAPIST: 'Okay, we accept that it is impossible for you to relax. But – just as an experiment, mind you – I want you to pretend you are relaxed. Pretend you don't have a worry in the world. Just pretend and act it out for ten minutes, that's all you have to do.'

> The subconscious cannot be bullied – through logic, willpower, common sense or any other mechanism – into behaving rationally. It must be *charmed* into reacting the way you want it to.

How long do you think it will be until our worrier is relaxed? Exactly. Ten minutes.

I hesitated before including this particular technique. My concern was that it may – like some of the other techniques in this book – appear too simplistic a solution for some of the cynics.

However, what may appear simplistic on the surface can still be effective. And this technique is just that.

It is based on the understanding that a great many – if not most – stresses and anxieties that affect us are not altogether rational. In other words, we worry about things that have passed, things that *might* be going to happen to us in the future, things that others *might* think of us now – as opposed to what *is*. Looked at in the cold light of day, those worries are not always very rational, are they?

Generally, these are products of the subconscious, rather than the conscious, mind. And sometimes the subconscious defies all rationality.

It follows, therefore, that if the subconscious is the instigator or nurturer of so many of your fears and anxieties, it might also be capable of being the alleviator.

But how? Is it possible to channel this force into a constructive therapeutic tool?

In an earlier chapter we discussed how the subconscious cannot be bullied – through logic, willpower, common sense or any other mechanism – into behaving rationally. That is not in its nature; that is not the way it works.

The subconscious must be *charmed* into reacting the way you want. This process of charming is the basis of all conditioning, hypnotism, rapport-building and habit formation. To be effective, the ideas you plant in it must appeal to the *imagination* rather than the intellect.

Enough theory. One of the most effective means available for influencing your subconscious was one you perfected at a very tender age. This technique allowed you to transcend the pains and drudgery of normal life, and could transport you into royal castles or distant galaxies in the blink of an eye.

I am writing, of course, of the ability to pretend.

Because it is creative and playful, and filled with unreal imagery, pretending is a powerful way to appeal to the subconscious. Some of the most skilled psychotherapists, particularly those who work with hypnosis, utilise this device to overcome the barriers and intrusions of the conscious mind. By having subjects *pretend* to be something or to feel a particular way, instead of actually trying to achieve it, they recruit the subject's subconscious in their efforts.

And this means success comes a hundred, a thousand times faster than if the conscious mind were trying to do it alone.

We can use such a technique to find instant peace and calm.

How it works

You're feeling anxious and tense. You know you've done all you can to address your problem, but still you're restless and uneasy. And as the minutes tick by, you grow uneasier and more anxious. You try telling yourself this is silly; that there is nothing you can do to vary what is happening, so you might as well not worry about it. You try to *force* yourself not to worry. But, of course, your worrying gets worse.

You would have been much calmer if you'd done this instead . . .

First of all, conjure up in your mind all the characteristics you would exhibit if you were a totally calm and relaxed person. You'd probably be lounging around with all the time in the world. Your gestures would be languid and almost lazy. Your breathing would be slow and deep. Your speech unhurried. Your lips would be slightly parted and there'd be the hint of a smile on your face. Your hands would be unclenched, your arms unfolded, your shoulders unhunched. Got the picture?

Now for the technique.

You simply *pretend* that you're feeling this way. You *pretend* that you carry yourself this way, that you're calm, relaxed and not concerned about a thing. *Pretend* you are in complete control of the situation, and every other situation like it. *Pretend* you're extremely familiar with this feeling of peace.

And, most important of all, **pretend that everybody else thinks you're this way all the time**.

Do this sincerely and diligently, and nothing is surer than you'll be believing it yourself in no time.

THE LET'S PRETEND TECHNIQUE

- Remember the Conditions of Calm.
- On your big screen conjure up an image of yourself as calm, relaxed and at peace with the world. Note your slow breathing, unclenched hands and teeth, the hint of a smile, languid gestures, the unhurried speech.
- Start pretending you are exactly like that. (This is only make-believe, so be as extreme as you like in these pretensions.) Flaunt how calm and relaxed you are.
- Now, most importantly, pretend that others see you being exactly the way you're pretending to feel.
- Spend the rest of your day, the rest of your life, even, pretending – only good can come of it.

The Calm Touch

You've heard about Pavlov's dog. As an experiment, each time he fed his dog, he sounded a bell. After some time of this, Pavlov could sound the bell and his dog would salivate in anticipation of being fed – there was no need to produce the food to arouse the reaction.

What's that got to do with making you feel calm?

Nothing, other than it is a well-known example of a pattern – known as a 'programmed conditioned response' – you can use to find immediate release from stress and anxiety.

A powerful example of this response is the Calm Touch. Before you attempt it, however, there are two guidelines to bear in mind:

a the time to *perfect* the Calm Touch is when you're calm;
b the time to *apply* it is when you're stressed.

The basis of the Calm Touch is the understanding that you can trigger a calming response in yourself – almost instantly – just by touching one specific part of your body in a certain way.

You might choose to press the inside of your left wrist with your right forefinger. You might choose to interlink the fingers of both hands. You might choose to pinch the top of your right thumbnail with your left hand. There is no magic to where you touch or how you touch. All that is important is that this touch, this trigger, is reasonably distinctive from your day-to-day list of scratchings, rubbings and gestures.

In the following section I will explain how to *program* a relaxing response into this touch. Once you have done this – and it needs to be done only once – all you will ever have to do is reproduce this touch and the response will be triggered. And you will be relaxed!

Sounds too easy to be effective? It just so happens to be a favoured tool of one of the world's fastest-growing schools of psychotherapeutic training. That's how well it works!

If you doubt that a once-only programming session is sufficient to take you through the rest of your life, try this simple experiment: recall one erotic experience from your past. Only one. One that you have never dared repeat, or succeeded in reproducing. Recall the details of it: what you were wearing, what the other party was wearing, the scents you could smell, the music or heavy breathing you could hear. Think back though all the feelings you felt at that time. The touches you experienced . . .

Getting aroused again? That is a classic example of a programmed condition response.

Preparation

Preparation is everything in the Calm Touch. Get this first part right and you can carry a powerful antidote to stress and tension – one that you can apply in any place, at any time.

Before you commence, give some thought to a time in your past when you felt totally calm and at peace with yourself and the world. You may have to go right back into your childhood – but somewhere in your past is an experience or an event that made you feel this way.

Take the time to find a powerful example now, because this is the key to the Calm Touch. (If you can't recall one that makes you feel good, postpone this exercise to another day. Sooner or later you will think of one.)

Yes, it's another 'big screen' exercise.

Taking that event from your past, 'see' yourself up on that screen participating, reliving it. Note as much detail as possible – what the light is like, what you're wearing, the colours of the surroundings.

Next, 'hear' all the sounds that are involved with that experience. Note them in detail.

Then, 'feel' what you were feeling then. The temperature of the day, the great sense of calm that flowed through your body. If you concentrate on these details sufficiently, that sense of calm will be flowing through your body once again.

When you believe you are re-experiencing that event to the fullest, apply a firm touch to some part of your body (you will need to have decided on this beforehand). Do it for a couple of seconds, then release it.

That is your Calm Touch. If you have performed those steps as prescribed to the best of your abilities, you will have programmed yourself to respond in the same way – that is, to feel totally calm and at peace – whenever that touch is applied.

Now, before you move on, sit quietly and apply your Calm Touch a couple of times just to prove to yourself that it works.

Application

From now on, each time you feel stressed or anxious, simply stop for a moment and apply the Calm Touch. That's all it should take to get those feelings of calm and peace flooding back.

You can do this anywhere. Sitting at your desk, in the back seat of a cab, in the dentist's waiting room. However, for maximum effectiveness, try to find a place that is quiet and free from distraction. The quieter it is, the better the Calm Touch will work.

THE CALM TOUCH

- Remember the Conditions of Calm.
- Recall an event from your past where you felt totally calm and at peace with yourself and the world.
- On your big screen, 'see' yourself participating, reliving that experience. Note the details – the light, your clothes, the colours of the surroundings. 'Hear' the sounds. 'Feel' the experience.
- When you're fully involved in the experience, apply a distinctive touch or pressure to one part of your body. Release it after a few seconds.
- Test that your Calm Touch is programmed as intended. Before you move, apply it a couple of times and notice the feeling of calm and peace come flooding back.
- Apply the Calm Touch whenever you're stressed or anxious. Preferably, do it somewhere quiet and free from distraction.

16

THE PHILOSOPHY OF CALM

There is a man I have shared seminar stages with who has dedicated much of his life to teaching people ways of dealing with stress. When pressed for the secret that allows him to stay cool in the most difficult situations, he confesses that it is largely philosophical.

'There are two guidelines I try to apply to all worrying situations,' he said. 'The first is that I refuse to lose sleep over minor issues. The second is that all issues are minor issues.'

Imagine if we could all think that way.

With one simple shift of attitude, most of the ills and misfortunes of our lives – excluding, of course, genuine tragedies and disasters – would simply vanish.

Following are a number of techniques which, through subtle shifts in focus or attitude, can immediately help you deal with the pressures and tensions of your everyday life.

The Universal Perspective

Most problems in life are either enhanced or diminished according to your perspective.

The threat of being fired from your job is greatly diminished the moment you have a better offer from another employer. A stern word from the woman in your life is nowhere near as shattering after ten years of marriage as it would be on a first date. The slight double chin you've been worrying about suddenly vanishes from your consciousness the moment you enter a room full of sumo wrestlers. The hunger you've been feeling because of a missed breakfast simply disappears when you're in the company of starving Rwandans.

Why? Because perspective is what colours the situations you face.

The exercise that follows – appropriated from a meditation seminar I once attended – is a simple way of changing your perspective when you're suffering from anxiety or a problem. The technique does not require you to think about your worry specifically, but to observe yourself where you are at that moment, then in your mind simply to change the perspective.

You can do this exercise anywhere. It only takes a minute or so to complete.

With eyes closed, visualise yourself sitting in the chair you're sitting in. Notice the clothes you're wearing, the way you're holding your hands. Notice these things as if you were a detached camera.

Now widen your perspective. See yourself in relation to the whole room. Note the placement of the furniture.

Then take 'the camera' outside the house. You can see the window of the room you're sitting in. You can see how the garden fits snugly around the house.

Wider now. You can see your house in relation to the whole street. A balloonist's perspective. You can see your neighbour's place, the restaurant on the corner, the traffic lights at the end of the street.

Much higher now.

Your street is a simple line passing through a suburb. There's the highway to the left, another suburb to the right.

Now the city is just a sea of twinkling lights along the coast.

An astronaut's perspective. Down there in the cloud haze is a swirl of brown and green which is the continent you live on. The Earth is just a globe. A shining, beautiful globe, rotating serenely in space . . .

The Earth is just a light in the heavens . . . A speck in our galaxy . . .

From here, your problems are so irrelevant, they hardly exist.

(After you have done this exercise once or twice, you can go straight to the Universal Perspective. It can be very fast, and very powerful.)

THE UNIVERSAL PERSPECTIVE

- Remember the Conditions of Calm. Sit in a comfortable chair. Remove your shoes. Rest your hands apart, comfortably on your lap.
- Form a picture of yourself in your mind. Do it as if you're a camera, completely detached. Note what you're wearing, the expression on your face, the way you're sitting.
- Now 'see' yourself in relation to the whole room. Note furniture placement, where you're sitting in the room.
- Your 'camera' is now positioned above the house. You can see the house in relation to the garden and surroundings.
- From a balloonist's point of view, 'see' your house in relation to the whole street. Then 'see' the street in relation to the suburb, and the suburb in relation to the city.
- Now you have an astronaut's view of the city as a speck on a beautiful coastline.
- And the Earth as a wonderful globe floating serenely in space.
- The Earth as a light among many planets.
- And as a speck in our galaxy.
- Hold this perspective, until your problem diminishes.

The Ten-year Plan

The technique that follows is conceptually similar to the Universal Perspective but does not depend so much on visualisation.

For this exercise, instead of placing a *visual* perspective on your problem, you choose a more abstract one – a *time* perspective.

The idea is to think back ten years – imagine yourself as you were at that time – then imagine how important your present problem would have seemed then. Almost invariably it will seem less important.

Now, think *forward* ten years from today. Try to imagine how important your present problem or anxiety will appear then. Once again, it will seem less important, less threatening.

The simplicity of this technique belies its effectiveness in putting the present into perspective. Try it; it works.

THE TEN-YEAR PLAN

- Remember the Conditions of Calm.
- Try to imagine what you were like exactly ten years ago. Recall the details: what you were wearing, how you wore your hair, where you lived, the attitudes you held.
- Imagine how that person of *ten years ago* would say if s/he knew how you were reacting to today's situation. Imagine how today's problems would have seemed then.
- Now, imagine what you'll be like in ten years' time. Note what you'll be wearing, the attitudes you'll have.
- Imagine how you'll view today's problem then.
- Pause, with these impressions, while your problem or anxiety diminishes or disappears.

Staying in the Present

At the root of most emotional disorders or discomforts is one of two conditions: concerns about the past, or anxiety about the future.

Scary, isn't it, how so much pain can be produced by states that simply do not exist. Both past and future are abstract concepts yet, in Western countries, concerns for what's past and what's yet to happen cause more insecurity, anxiety, fear, frustration and tension than anything that ever really happens.

People who carry concerns about the past – such as guilt, regret or embarrassment – are concerned with something they have no hope of influencing. Similarly, people who have anxiety about the future – whether they'll ever be safe, happy, loved or successful – are generally concerned with something they can have only minor influence over, at best.

The only state you can really influence is the present.

Will Rogers was once asked what he'd do if he only had five days left to live. 'Why,' he answered matter-of-factly, 'I'd live each day one at a time.'

Basic, but profound.

Have you ever secretly envied those people whose lives seem to be an ongoing game or adventure, who are always striving to have a good time, who continually seem to live for the present? Have you ever worried that the conservative ideals of your upbringing – planning for the future, saving, working for retirement – severely limit your capacity to enjoy and get the most out of life?

Most happy, contented people recognise that the ideal is a midway course between the two extremes. Most worriers do not.

The people who are most calm and relaxed about their lives are not those who have unblemished or uncomplicated pasts, nor are they those who have sorted out everything to do with their futures. *They are those who have learned to live in the present.* (Note, 'in' the present, not 'for' the present.)

This state is astoundingly easy to achieve.

Take a lesson from your children: watch how the smallest child lives every moment for the pleasure of that moment; watch how they become totally engrossed in the pattern on the carpet, or the

THE ANTIDOTE TO BOREDOM

Boredom is one of life's most common stressors. When you are frustrated by the lack of anything satisfying to do, your tension levels escalate.

The antidote to this condition is exquisitely simple.

If you concentrate wholly on whatever you have to do – however mundane or meaningless it may appear – time flies, and you derive satisfaction from your efforts.

If you immerse yourself totally in a task, so that you achieve the very best result you are capable of, you will find that task becomes almost like meditation in itself. (Indeed, this is the 'Little Way' made famous by St Thérèse of Lisieux.)

Not only is this the antidote to boredom, it is a sure way to become calm and relaxed.

switch on the video recorder. Notice how calm a child is at that moment?

To duplicate this calm, all you have to do is concentrate on living each moment to the fullest.

Concentrate your attention and appreciation on getting the most out of every second. If you're eating, savour every bite, be aware of every texture and taste as if you'd never experienced anything of their kind before; savour the subtlety of the scents, colours and arrangement on the plate. (Incidentally, this is a great way to get your weight under control as well.)

If you devote your attention completely to the eating – not to planning tomorrow's work schedule or trying to remember how you varied the recipe last time you cooked it – you will appreciate it more than ever before. More importantly, though, you will have discovered a technique for achieving true peace and calm.

Whether you're eating, weeding, driving or playing, if you concentrate on doing it to the fullest, if your attention is centred on what you are doing – that is, on the present – you will become calm.

It's as simple as that.

17

CALM PHYSICALS

We have already established that most anxieties and stress-related problems are a product of what is inside your head as opposed to what happens to your body and, as such, are more logically remedied by 'internal' techniques.

Even so, many sufferers are not all that comfortable with the 'mumbo jumbo' techniques that deal primarily with the emotions and the subconscious. These people find comfort in physical, tangible, more demonstrable solutions.

Fortunately, there is a whole range of physical measures that are extremely efficient in reversing the effects of negative stress. We have already covered a number of them.

Foremost among these is physical exercise. As it is probably the most beneficial way of burning off excess 'stress chemicals' accumulated in our bodies, almost any physical exercise will reduce the ill-effects of stress.

Following is a variety of physical techniques that do one of two things: either they directly counter the effects of negative stress – Calm Exercises (pages 73–82) and the Power Breathing technique (pages 65–9) fall into this category – or they reverse the *physical* processes that lead to stress.

The Jaw Release

One of the most common manifestations of stress is the clamped jaw and clenched teeth. It's estimated that 25 per cent of the population are jaw clenchers. Yet, even if you are one of these, there is every possibility you will not have noticed: because the condition is ever-present.

This does not lessen its impact, however. Taut upper jaw muscles lead to clenched teeth – or vice versa – then spread through your shoulder/neck/head area until you're feeling tense overall. (See 'Headache' on page 29.)

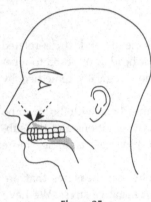

Worse, tense jaw muscles have a habit of spreading their havoc throughout the body; indeed, some therapists claim that a variety of chronic back problems stem from this habit.

These days, it is not uncommon for dentists to provide little devices called 'splints' or 'de-programmers' (see page 222) for their patients who complain of headache or other problems that stem

Figure 25

from clenching the teeth. Although simple in design, these dental prosthetics are extremely effective at reducing muscular tension in the jaw area. Their drawback is they need to be professionally fitted and, as a result, can turn out to be expensive.

The Jaw Release is a better, faster and cheaper solution. And it will take effect almost immediately.

It works like this: lightly press the tongue against the roof of your mouth (Figure 25), just behind the front teeth. That's all you do. As long as you maintain that light pressure, your lower jaw muscles (masseter muscles) will be relaxed. This, in turn, encourages a reduction in tension in the upper jaw (internal and external pterygoid muscles) and still farther into the area around the temples (temporalis muscle).

So much long-lasting relief from just pressing your tongue lightly against the roof of your mouth!

Here's another technique that works on the same problem.

Open your mouth, slowly, as wide as you can without strain. Then close. Repeat this for about two minutes.

JAW RELEASE 1

- First become aware of the tension in your jaw. Clench your jaw tighter, then release it.
- Lightly press the tongue against the roof of the mouth – behind the front teeth. Allow your lips to part slightly. Feel your jaw muscles relax.
- Repeat this exercise several times a day, particularly at night before falling asleep.

Next, press your fist under your chin and apply light pressure. Then, opening your mouth, press your jaw downwards against this resistance – not too hard or you'll get cramp.

Maintain this pressure for about a minute.

If you repeat this exercise several times throughout the day, you will prevent jaw clenching from taking serious effect.

JAW RELEASE 2

- Slowly open your mouth as wide as you can without strain. Close. Repeat for about 2 minutes.
- Lightly press your fist under your chin. Opening your mouth, press your jaw downwards against your fist.
- Maintain this pressure for about a minute. Repeat the exercise throughout the day.

Lotus Hands

Ask the average novelist for the most visible sign of stress in a character and she will say 'The hands'. This is why novelists write about wringing hands, clasped fingers, white knuckles, clenched fists and so on. Are these just dreadful clichés, or are they really the most visible signs of stress in a person?

Okay, they are dreadful clichés – but they are also the most visible signs of stress.

More than that, however, such actions actually spread tension throughout the body. Tightly clasped hands lead to tense arm muscles, lead to tense back muscles, lead to who knows what.

It follows, therefore, that if you relieve this tension in your hands, you can relieve it in other parts of your body as well. You will be surprised at how powerful this technique can really be.

There are three simple ways of easing the tension from your wrists, hands and fingers. All of them are common to the various forms of meditation or yoga.

Before you perform them, unfold your arms and loosen the muscles.

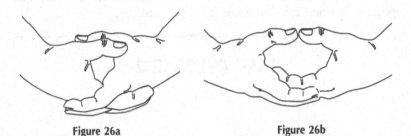

Figure 26a   Figure 26b

The first technique is one you would have seen in the movies when a yogi sits in the full lotus position. Each hand rests on a knee, palms turned up, thumbtips barely touching the fingertips (middle and ring fingers) of each hand. This technique is said to be effective on both physical and cosmic levels, although it may look a little contrived when you do it in public. But it works!

The second technique may also appear a little contrived but it, too, is worth remembering because it works so well. All you do is gently rest the thumbtips and fingertips of one hand against the corresponding thumbtips and fingertips of the other. No pressure; just the lightest touch.

The last technique works equally as well, but is one you can perform in public – standing on the bus queue, sitting at your desk or waiting for the dentist to call your name. Its beauty is the way it relates to the clenched hands (Figure 26a) of a tense person.

To effect it, all you have to do is first clasp your fingers tightly, unclasp them, then nestle your left hand inside your right hand (Figure 26b) and let your thumbtips touch.

Do this as lightly as is physically possible. Concentrate on doing it perfectly.

At first, this will feel a little awkward and you will feel the urge to press your hands tightly together. Persist, the urge passes after thirty seconds or so.

LOTUS HANDS

- Unfold your arms and shake them out so the muscles feel more relaxed.
- Clasp the fingers, tightly, then unclasp them – so you become aware of what tension feels like.
- Disentwine the fingers, then nestle your left hand inside your right. Let the thumbtips touch, *gently*.
- Remain like this as long as you would normally remain with clasped fingers.
- Perform other calm techniques while Power Breathing.

The Calm Demeanour

Remember the scenario we covered in an earlier section?

WORRIER: 'I find it impossible to relax. I've tried every technique, but I still find it impossible to relax.'
THERAPIST: 'Okay, we accept that it is impossible for you to relax. But just as an experiment, mind you – I want you to *pretend* you are relaxed. Pretend you don't have a worry in the world. Just pretend and act it out for ten minutes, that's all you have to do.'

Tighten your forehead and eyebrows into a frown, an ugly frown. Keep frowning until they hurt.

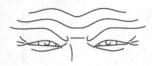

Now raise your eyebrows and feel the tension lift.

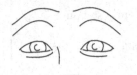

From a pretending point of view alone, the Calm Demeanour is a powerful technique. But that is only part of its power; its real strength comes from distinct physiological changes that you produce in your own body.

It is also one of the most easily accomplished techniques in this book.

Negative stress effects some of its most painful and noticeable work around the head and neck areas of the body. A tense face is instantly recognisable. The muscles constrict in all possible directions: the jaw is clenched, the forehead furrowed, eyebrows knotted, eyes slightly squinted, teeth gritted and the lips pulled tightly shut. (Equally pronounced are the taut neck muscles, spreading their tension into the cranium, down through the shoulders, into the back. However, these can be treated with yet another technique.)

By reversing those physical characteristics, you can create a sense of calm for yourself.

Start with the forehead and eyebrows which, when you're tense, are tight and knotted. Releasing the tension here has an immediate positive effect. And it is so easy to achieve. Simply raise the eyebrows – subtly, almost imperceptably to an onlooker – and the tension will be lifted! Try it; you'll be surprised at how much difference such a small action can make. The object, however, is to go about with your eyebrows *slightly* lifted.

Next, we come to the clenched teeth and taut jaw muscles. By relaxing these two areas, you will also be heading towards a state of relaxation.

How do you do this? Simply press your tongue against the roof of your mouth as we covered in the Jaw Release.

Finally, we come to the remainder of the facial muscles – the site of so much tension. Once again, the technique for relaxing these is beautifully simple. It is also one you've been using yourself since childhood.

It's a smile.

The simple act of smiling relaxes *all* those facial muscles that stress tightens. Moreover, studies now show that certain types of smile (the genuine, 'wrinkly-eyed' variety) actually stimulate the pleasure centres of the brain. In other words, this kind of smile triggers a feeling of happiness without any further input. Try it. The effect is immediate.

To effect maximum relaxation of the tense facial muscles, tighten your lips as far as possible, then relax them into a smile.

THE CALM DEMEANOUR

- Frown, then raise the eyebrows in a slightly exaggerated fashion. Do this a few times until your eyebrows and forehead area feel relaxed.
- Press the tongue lightly against the roof of the mouth, just behind the front teeth – until your teeth unclench and your jaw muscles relax.
- Smile. Tighten your lips then relax them into a smile. Do this several times to relax your facial muscles.
- Be aware of how it feels to have your forehead, jaw and facial muscles totally relaxed. Practise carrying that feeling about with you.

Calm Postures

Your posture not only reflects the way you feel, but also influences it. Slumped shoulders, dropped chin and folded arms inhibit your ability to breathe deeply which, in turn, affects the way you handle stress and tension. Clenched fingers spread tension into the hands, up the arms, into the shoulders and back.

Worse, such posture often influences your state of mind as well as making you feel negative and under threat. (If you doubt that appearances affect the way you feel, remember that walk around the block: if you do it proudly, chin up, shoulders back, looking people squarely in the eye it will leave you with a significantly better feeling than if you walk around with your shoulders stooped, head down, feet shuffling.)

As we have demonstrated with earlier techniques, altering your physical situation can change the way you feel. Moreover, it can do so almost instantly.

In their most basic form, the Calm Postures reverse the postures you adopt when you are under stress. By simply lifting your chin, straightening your spine, pulling back your shoulders, unclasping your fingers, you can make yourself feel more relaxed – it's as easy as that.

However, many highly stressed people will discover that, by adopting the above measures, they will only partially achieve the objective. Because when you're under pressure, you lose touch with what's 'normal'. Your idea of

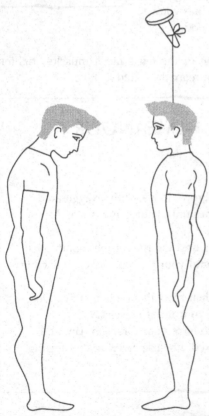

Figure 27

straight spine, lifted chin and so on will probably not look all that different to your stressed posture. And, if someone were to help you into the correct posture, you would say it felt unnatural.

The Calm Postures employ an ingenious aid for effecting a stress-free posture. It is a length of shiny, unbreakable piano wire.

What makes this piano wire useful is the fact that it 'attaches' to the centre of your head and has the capacity to 'lift' you.

Of course, the piano wire I am referring to is imaginary. You *imagine* it being attached to the top of your head; you *imagine* it lifting your body so that you are almost suspended above the ground (Figure 27). You will feel your body straighten in a way that, at first, may seem slightly unnatural. It is, however, simply correct posture.

This is how your body was designed to stand. And to sit. By adopting this posture, you will breathe better, you will feel less constricted and you will feel calmer. Combine it with the Power Breathing techniques earlier in this book and you have a powerful calming combination that can be put into effect at any time in any place.

CALM POSTURES

- Unclasp fingers, unfold arms, pull the shoulders back and lift your chin.
- Imagine a shiny, strong length of piano wire attached to the top of your skull and connected to the ceiling.
- 'Tighten' this wire until you are almost 'suspended' above the ground. Feel your body stretch out all the way up your backbone.
- When you feel comfortable with this straightened posture, commence Power Breathing.
- Remain in this position for several minutes.
- Use this technique whenever you're standing, sitting, driving or walking for extended periods.

The Calm Unfold

When you feel tense, your body is warning you that it is suffering the ill-effects of stress.

You feel it tightening in the back of your neck. Stiffening. Dragging up into the back of your cranium. You feel it tightening across your shoulders – down low between your shoulder blades and up to the base of your neck. Even your posture changes: the shoulders are lifted and brought forward. You feel it in your lower back where the tension concentrates. You feel it as a constriction in your chest wall. And in your abdominal muscles. You feel it in your clenched fingers.

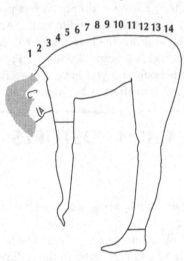

Figure 28

Stress and tension work their way through your body, from the base of your skull, through your shoulders, all the way down to your buttocks. And it is all unnecessary because it can be prevented so very easily.

The Calm Unfold is a simple exercise. It is designed to loosen all those tightening muscles and, *combined with other techniques*, will instil a sense of calm almost immediately.

Stand upright. Imagine that piano wire attached to your cranium, lifting you towards the ceiling.

When you are comfortable with your upright position, drop your chin to your chest. Then, one vertebra at a time, begin to roll your spine forward, breathing out as you do so. Let your shoulders drop. Let your chest roll forward.

Keep 'rolling' until your entire upper body hangs limply. Shoulders, arms, wrists and fingers relaxed and dangling (Figure 28).

Stay like this as long as it feels comfortable.

The next stage is the reverse of that action. Unrolling one vertebra at a time, come back to the upright position.

THE CALM UNFOLD

- Stand upright, Power Breathing. Imagine a thin piano wire attached to your cranium, lifting you towards the ceiling.
- Drop your chin to your chest.
- Then, one vertebra at a time, 'roll' your spine until your whole upper body hangs limply towards the floor. Breathe out as you do so. Your shoulders, arms, wrists and fingers will be relaxed and dangling.
- Stay in this position as long as it feels comfortable. Try for a few minutes, but if you feel any pressure, go immediately to the next step.
- Reverse the procedure until you are upright again. Repeat this as many times as it takes until your neck, shoulder and back muscles are relaxed.

Unfold with Chair

In *extreme* cases of tension and anxiety, it may be necessary for you to employ techniques that demand no effort on your part at all. The exercise that follows is one such technique.

It is similar to the Calm Unfold in that it releases the muscular tensions in the neck, shoulders and back. But, unlike the Calm Unfold, it requires virtually no thought or conscious effort on your part. (It's a technique sometimes recommended in severe asthma cases.)

How easy is it?

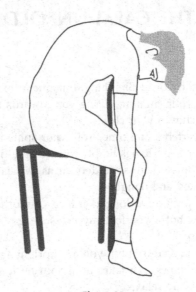

Figure 29

Take a straight-backed chair. Sit facing backwards on it. Make sure your feet are slightly apart and flat on the floor. Then drape your arms and shoulders loosely over the chair back. Let your hands dangle loosely. Free your fingers. Let your head hang freely. At the same time, ensure that your breathing is deep and diaphragmatic (Power Breathing).

That's all you have to do. Easy?

While you may feel a little strange sitting backwards on a chair like this, it's amazing how quickly this technique works in helping you breathe evenly, and in releasing tension from your shoulders, back and neck. And, once the tension is released from these areas, you can use any of the other techniques in this book to enhance this feeling of calm.

UNFOLD WITH CHAIR

- Remember the Conditions of Calm. Commence slow Power Breathing. Continue for at least 1 minute.
- Sit backwards on a straight-backed chair. Drape your arms and shoulders over its back; let them hang loosely. Let all your tensions dissolve into that chair. Ensure your breathing is deep and diaphragmatic.
- Stay in this position as long as it feels comfortable.
- When you feel more relaxed, employ other techniques from this book.

Feet Up Technique

Here's something else you can do with a chair.

The Feet Up Technique is one taught to me by a masseur; he didn't like to tell too many of his clients about it as it denied him a source of business.

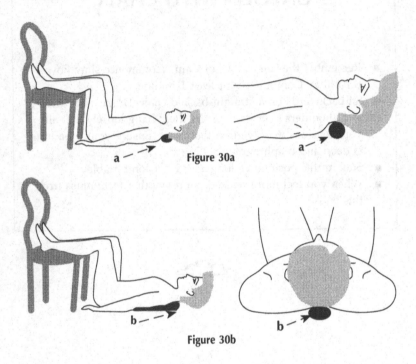

Figure 30a

Figure 30b

It is a simple, practical way of finding relief from the tensions that build up in your back and neck muscles. Moreover, it is about as lazy a technique as you are ever likely to encounter.

The Feet Up Technique requires nothing more of you but to lie there on the floor with – you guessed it – your feet up on a chair. That's all. Not only is it relaxing in itself, but it also removes strain from the lower back.

However, that's only part of the story. The rest involves a small towel (a hand towel or small bath towel, whichever feels more comfortable to you). There are two ways to use it.

If tension gathers more in your neck than your back muscles, place the towel behind your neck at the base of your skull as you lie on the floor (Figure 30a). You will feel a little pressure against those tense muscles. The more tense you are, the more uncomfortable this will initially feel. (If you find yourself getting dizzy or nauseous, remove the towel.) Remember, though, you are *meant* to feel some pressure – that is what releases the tension.

If there is more tension in your back muscles than your neck, place the rolled towel *down* the length of your back so a shoulder blade falls on either side of it (Figure 30b).

Remain in that reclining position for 10–20 minutes while you continue Power Breathing.

FEET UP TECHNIQUE

- Remember the Conditions of Calm.
- Lie on your back on the floor, with your feet resting on a chair.
- If your neck muscles are tense, take a rolled towel and place it behind your neck at the base of your skull (a). Use a hand towel or small bath towel, depending on what you find comfortable. Remember, though, you are *meant* to feel a little pressure – but if you feel dizzy or nauseous, desist.
- If it is your *back* muscles that contain the tension, take a rolled towel and place it down the length of your back (b). Allow a shoulder blade to fall on either side of it.
- Stay in this position for at least 10–20 minutes. Perform Power Breathing exercises.
- When you feel more relaxed, employ other techniques from this book.

Calm Hug

One of the most effective techniques for finding comfort in troubled moments is one you already
know about. In fact, it is fundamental to the wellbeing of all
humans.

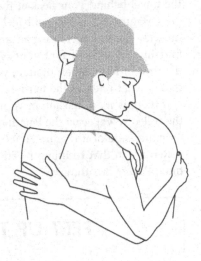

It's the act of touching.

Not only has touching been
with us since birth, but it is a necessary part of every individual's
psychological development. It's
instinctive, it builds self-esteem
and it makes the recipient – as
well as the giver – feel needed and
valued.

And, in accordance with the
theme of this book, it helps both the giver and the receiver to relax.

Observe how the embrace of a parent soothes an upset child. Notice
how, in moments of trauma, you will so readily fall into another person's embrace. Notice how a kiss or a handshake takes the sting out
of an argument.

If you can overcome the barriers to intimacy that so many people
suffer, if you can touch and be touched by another – especially in a
non-sexual way – you will know one of life's greatest secrets to calm
and relaxation.

There is no mystery to the Calm Hug. Go up to someone you know
and trust and throw your arms around them. If you feel uncomfortable
about doing this, warn them first. Say, 'I need a hug; do you mind?'

Then just hold on and wait for the sense of calm and wellbeing that
accompanies it. Cling. Soak up the warmth and humanity. Enjoy the
physical communication, knowing full well that the other person is
getting as much out of it as you are.

And, most important of all, do it often.

Do it daily. Do it hourly. Do it as frequently as you can.

The Dance

Most of the techniques in *Instant Calm* require you to turn off the radio, be still, and seek peace and quiet. This one requires you to turn on the music, turn it up loud, and jump about a like a mad person.

Of course we are speaking about dance.

Dance works on two quite separate levels. The first and most obvious is the physical: the sheer, full-bore exercise of it is guaranteed to distract even the most dedicated worrier. The second is psychological, and even more effective: the creative, physical expression of what you're hearing (the music) is a fast and sure way to distance yourself from stress.

Any type of dancing will work – as long as it's not so structured that you cannot throw yourself wholeheartedly into it. Creative, free-form dancing is one of the fastest and most powerful ways of ridding yourself of stress and taking your mind off your woes.

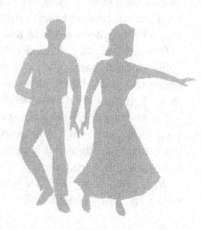

For some, it can work more reliably than any other form of stress release. And, for some, it will certainly be more fun. But what about those who hate dancing?

If you fall into this category, perhaps you should consider this technique even more so, because those who 'hate' dancing usually happen to be the worrying Type A personality grouping. And if you can give yourself over to the rhythm and let yourself go, dance works even better for Type A people than it does for committed dancers.

Forget about how clumsy you might be, and about who might be watching; just turn up the music and let yourself go.

Orgasm

We may not always recognise the fact, but so many of the pressures and tensions of everyday life are sexually oriented. Or at least fanned by sexual drives.

Most people will deny this, of course. And, true, for most people these forces are subtle, maybe not even noticeable. But they are there. Building. Adding to tension.

How do you relieve it? Have an orgasm. Or two.

Yoga

One cannot write a book on calm without mentioning yoga. Hatha yoga is an ancient and most satisfying way of controlling the emotions and achieving deep levels of relaxation.

Through a rigidly defined combination of movements, breath and bodily control, hatha yoga not only paves the way for physical and emotional peace, but is also reputedly a path to spiritual enlightenment. You can only determine this for yourself, of course.

Try as I've done, I have not succeeded in simplifying the traditional yoga techniques into a suitable (that is, fast-operating) format for this book. I have mentioned it here because many find it an important step in the search for true calm.

With hatha yoga, there are no shortcuts. The study is a serious and time-consuming commitment.

The Rocker

Psychologists I've consulted in preparing this book have failed to agree on why the following technique works. I'm not sure why myself – but it does work.

People grieving or suffering great trauma do it intuitively. Grandmothers in the old days used to do it intuitively. Parents do it intuitively when their babies are upset.

It's rocking.

For reasons on which we can only speculate, the rocking motion is a wonderfully soothing palliative for emotional suffering. Especially if you're suffering from anxiety or stress. Perhaps it has something to do with the expenditure of energy; perhaps it is something more primal, that relates back to the time in the womb (which most of us have experienced at least once in our lives).

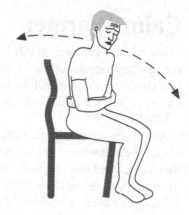

Figure 31

Whatever the rationale, a great many people find instant relief the moment they start using it. And, as it doesn't require any training or special effort, what have you go to lose?

How do you do it?

Sit in a straight-backed chair, Power Breathing. Wrap your arms about yourself (don't fold them), and start rocking back and forth from the waist up.

Don't be deceived by the simplicity. This technique works, even if we don't understand the reasons for it.

THE ROCKER

- Sit in a straight-backed chair, Power Breathing.
- Wrap your arms about yourself. Wrap them, don't fold them.
- Start rocking backwards and forwards, slowly, from the waist up.

Calm Warmer

Many of the techniques in this book are little more than a reversal of the physical manifestations of stress. If you are a sufferer of tension, one characteristic you will be familiar with is cold hands: the more tense you are, the colder your hands will be.

Why is this so?

At stressful moments, the fight or flight syndrome mentioned earlier causes the following responses: your adrenal glands release 'stress hormones' (epinephrine and norepinephrine) into the bloodstream which, in turn, increase your heart rate and blood pressure, as well as constricting the blood vessels in your digestive system and skin. At the same time your breathing becomes shallow; this reduces the amount of carbon dioxide in your bloodstream, which upsets your blood's pH (acid–alkaline levels) balance, which can cause too much calcium to rush into muscles and nerves.

This will eventually result in your fingers and toes feeling tingly and cold. It follows, therefore, that if you could reverse this condition, you would start to feel calmer.

CALM WARMER

- Rub your hands together furiously until they start to 'burn'.
- Stop, and let them hang loosely. Gently rotate them in a clockwise, then anti-clockwise direction, 5 times each way.
- Drag the backs of your hands against each other, backwards and forwards. Do this 10 times, very gently, the skin barely touching.
- Slowly brush the back of each hand with the backs of your fingernails in an upwards motion. Do this as gently as you can, 10 times with each hand.
- Follow with other calming techniques.

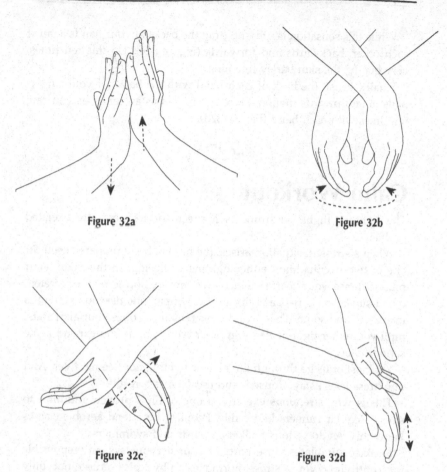

Figure 32a

Figure 32b

Figure 32c

Figure 32d

In bio-feedback, you can relieve tension and even migraine headaches simply by concentrating your attention on raising the temperature in your hands. The Calm Warmer does this through physical means.

On the surface, this may seem like an overly simplistic solution to a complex problem. It may be simple, but it does work.

To begin with, all you have to do is rub your hands together, furiously, until they're hot (Figure 32a). This may take a minute or so. When your hands are 'burning', stop and dangle them towards the floor (Figure 32b). Gently rotate them in a clockwise, then anti-clockwise motion, five times each way. You will feel your fingers tingling.

While this sensation is present, drag the backs of your hands against each other, backwards and forwards (Figure 32c). Do this ten times, very gently, the skin barely touching.

Finally, brush the back of each hand with the backs of your finger-nails in an upwards motion. Once again, do this as gently as you can, ten times with each hand (Figure 32d).

Calm Workout

The fight or flight syndrome is a precursor to most stress-related problems.

When a stressful situation arises, the human body prepares itself for one of two eventualities: either fighting or fleeing. In this state, your muscles tense, your heart rate increases, anxiety hormones are secreted, blood sugar levels rise, activity in the sympathetic nervous system is increased, and so on. These conditions remain, as does your alert state, until you either fight or flee – in other words, until you expend some serious energy.

Yet most of us go through life neither fighting nor fleeing. Ever. And our stress levels stay aroused, and escalate, as a result.

This is why strenuous exercise is one of life's proven antidotes to stress. Regular runners know this. People who attend aerobic classes know this. As do serious walkers, cyclists and swimmers.

Exercise stimulates those parts of your nervous system responsible for controlling your 'stress hormones'. Physical exercise not only reduces these chemicals in your body – calming the nerves, inducing a restful feeling, helping you to sleep better – but also enhances your long-term ability to deal with stress and stressful situations.

One note of caution: although marathon runners and 'gym addicts' might deny this, obsessive or extreme forms of exercise can have the reverse effect and actually *increase* your stress levels.

Assuming you are not suffering any serious medical conditions (have a medical checkup if you're not sure) a relaxed ideal is three to five workouts a week, each at 70 per cent of your maximum heart rate, lasting for 20–30 minutes.

To calculate your maximum heart rate, subtract your age from 220.

Thus, if you're forty years old, your maximum heart rate is 180 beats per minute (220 − 40 = 180). Your ideal *exercise* pulse rate is 70 per cent of that maximum, or 126 beats per minute. To calculate your pulse rate at any time, place your fingertips on your pulse and count the number of beats in 60 seconds.

Naturally, if you have any existing medical conditions that may be affected by exercise you should consult your medical adviser before working out.

THE CALM WORKOUT

- Whenever you feel under pressure or suffering from anxiety, throw yourself into a strenuous physical activity.
- Using these timing guides as an example, do one of the following.
  - Walk briskly for 45 minutes.
  - Run for 25 minutes.
  - Swim for 25 minutes.
  - Cycle (at a reasonable speed) for 45 minutes.
  - Perform aerobics for 25 minutes.
  - Dance for 30–45 minutes.
- Do it at least three times a week and you will begin to build a resistance to stress and an on-going feeling of calm.

Golf

I urge you to exercise great caution when applying the following technique.

Although I have escaped the pitfalls relating to this therapy myself, I know of many previously level-headed people who have fallen victim to its lure. Indeed, many of its advocates have long since forfeited the right to be described as level-headed.

I am writing about golf.

In many ways, it has no equal as a relaxation therapy. Several hours of moderate exercise, often begun early in the morning, usually conducted out of doors, often accompanied by mindless prattle about the virtues of five irons and the trajectories of little balls.

The detail of how it works? I have no idea. All I know is that, for some, it works like no other therapy.

But please don't say you were not warned! Its calming benefits can be easily overshadowed by its addictiveness.

18

CALM PRESSURES

One of the oldest and most time-proven means of relaxation and relieving tension is that brought about through touch.

While massage in its various forms, acupressure, chiropractic and reflexology are some of the better-known stress-relief therapies, even the most basic forms of touching can be beneficial. You have been conscious of this since birth.

Naturally, the trained practitioners of these disciplines will have considerably more to offer than the condensed offerings included in this book. Nevertheless, the simplified techniques that follow will allow you to avail yourself of many of the benefits of these natural therapies without having to run off to a masseur or reflexologist every time you feel under stress.

The Calm Pressure techniques are derived from the four broad disciplines that follow.

Massage

Massage has been one of the growth industries of the Eighties. Whereas at first many saw it in a sensual context, massage is now known for the powerful remedial qualities it possesses.

The three most common areas of massage are Swedish, Shiatsu and Deep Tissue (which, as a form of Visceral Healing Massage, is related to Shiatsu). Of the three, the last is the most complex and difficult to apply, so has been overlooked for the purpose of this book.

Both Swedish and Shiatsu have their roots in centuries-old healing traditions. They are designed to direct the blood flow to various parts of the body – to stimulate the heart, to encourage more oxygen into

the muscles (thus reducing aches and pains) and to encourage the elimination of toxins from the body.

However, it is what they achieve in stress relief that concerns us. At
the completion of a massage, you will be enjoying a unique state – a
combination of deep relaxation and energy: skin tingling, muscles
loose, and your mind at peace.

Swedish massage

Midway through the last century, a long-standing Swedish tradition of
massage was crystallised into a four-point system of 'manipulative
therapy'.

Despite various attempts by entrepreneurs to give it different brand
names over the years, Swedish massage remains fundamentally the
same. It is still the most widely known type of massage in use today.

Because it consists primarily stroking and kneading, and is performed with oils on naked flesh, Swedish massage is known more for
its pleasurable and sensual qualities than for its healing abilities. Yet
devotees believe regular massage treatments are as important to a good
state of health as are diet and exercise.

Swedish massage does require another participant, however. As far
as I can determine, none of its techniques are particularly effective –
nor particularly possible – when performed alone.

Shiatsu

Based on a field of Chinese medicine in use since the Tsin dynasty of
about 300 BC, and combined with the relatively modern discipline of
osteopathy, Japan's shiatsu is claimed to unblock the body's energy
channels (meridians or acupuncture points) thus relieving tension and
correcting other physiological ailments.

Shiatsu is sometimes considered to be a more 'spiritual' form of
massage than Swedish because it embraces the Eastern philosophy of
balance between mind and body, and because it demands a high level
of communication (non-verbal) between giver and receiver. As it
mainly involves pressures rather than stroking – using elbows and
knees, as well as hands – and is generally applied through loose
clothing, it is considered less sensual than its Western counterpart.

Its devotees, however, consider it to be superior in all but the most superficial respects. They believe it has vastly more effective healing and stress-relieving properties, and they also believe these to be longer-lasting. As well, shiatsu therapists are often expected to be intuitive about their clients' physiological state and stress levels.

Because much of shiatsu's power comes from downward pressures applied to certain points throughout the body, you can employ some of its techniques by yourself.

Acupressure

Even though shiatsu employs much of the knowledge derived from this Chinese art, acupressure is a different discipline altogether to both shiatsu and acupuncture (a development it precedes by centuries).

The Chinese have known for many centuries that pressing, tapping or massaging certain points of the body can bring relief from pain or illness. Even though there have been important developments to this art in recent times (such as ear acupressure, developed in 1957) the core techniques have remained fundamentally the same.

Of course, proficiency at acupressure requires many years of study and it would be foolish of us to believe that a few pages of *Instant Calm* are going to equal that. But these are techniques that can be extremely beneficial as long as you follow three important points: you must find the correct pressure point, apply movement in the correct direction, and employ the correct method and pressure.

Apply those three principles, and you'll find the acupressure techniques in this book will be both easy to follow and powerful in what they can achieve.

Reflexology

Although ancient texts show that Asians, Indians, Egyptians and even Russians used massage of the feet in order to promote health, the practice of reflexology is by no means ancient.

It was developed in the 1930s by physiologist Eunice Ingham and Dr William Fitzgerald (who also developed the concept of zone therapy which is covered below).

The principle behind reflexology is that areas of the feet correspond to energy channels which extend throughout the body. By applying pressures to specific places on the foot, a reflexologist strives to unblock energy channels – in a way not unlike that of a shiatsu practitioner – and thus bring relief from pain or illness. This is not surprising, considering reflexology's origins in Chinese medicine.

According to reflexology theory, the feet are mini-maps of the body and its organs. Because we keep our feet covered and protected, they are sensitive and particularly receptive to subtle treatment. Simply by applying pressures to specific areas of the 'foot map', therapists claim to be able to relieve problems in other parts of the body.

There is a practical side to all of this.

Massaging the feet stimulates more than 7000 nerve endings – this can clear neural pathways, facilitate deep relaxation and improve circulation, all of which help the body to function more efficiently.

Whatever the wider claims about reflexology's healing properties, it does work wonders in the area of stress relief and relaxation.

Better still, it is a treatment you can apply yourself.

Zone therapy

I came upon zone therapy quite by accident. In a search through the local library's health-oriented data base, I was intrigued by the name of Dr Lust. Dr Benedict Lust. Anyone with a name like that had to be worthy of further investigation. His book, *Zone Therapy*, was first published in 1928. Subsequent research has attributed this healing system to an American–Englishman, Dr William Fitzgerald.

Zone therapy is claimed to be more scientifically based than disciplines such as reflexology. The 'zones' on which it is based are the areas between the ten electromagnetic fields that cover the body. By applying pressures and stimulation to certain areas of the body, you are supposed to be able to treat other parts of the body (particularly the nervous system, organs and glands) in corresponding electromagnetic zones.

Zone therapy employs fingertip pressure, as well as stimulation by fingernails, combs, pencils, rubber bands and other colourful miscellaneous items.

19

FIRST PARTY PRESSURES

When you think about it, there should be no one better equipped to massage away your pains and stresses than yourself; after all, no one knows better than you where the sore spots are, what feels good, and what feels too painful.

Unfortunately, there are physical limitations to the healing, soothing pressures you can exert yourself: there is only so far you can reach, only so much pressure you can apply, only so much relaxation you can derive when you're doing all the work yourself.

Even so, there are techniques you can employ that work very successfully indeed. Following are some of the more effective.

Digital Jaw Relaxer

Taut upper jaw muscles lead to clenched teeth – or vice versa – then 'refer' pain through your shoulder/neck/head area until you're feeling tense overall.

Quite a lot of damage from a tight jaw.

It follows, then, that a technique that can relieve the pressure in your jaw will help you to ease the feelings of tension that it promotes throughout the body. You can do this with the Digital Jaw Relaxer – a simple pressure technique that works quickly on the offending muscular area.

The Digital Jaw Relaxer requires only a modicum of skill. Using the tip of the index finger of each hand, apply pressure to the jaw muscle where it passes along the cheek by the earlobe. You will feel an

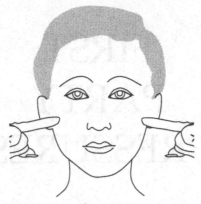

Figure 33

indentation, and the area will probably be quite tender. Apply pressure until a light pain can be felt in your jaw area. Maintain the pressure for about five seconds, then *slowly* release.

Repeat this exercise at least ten times. Pressure, release; pressure, release; pressure, release.

When the tension has eased, perform the Jaw Release exercise from pages 126–7.

DIGITAL JAW RELAXER

- Place the tip of the index finger against the jaw muscle that runs down the cheek by the earlobe. You will feel an indentation, and the area may be tender.
- Apply a direct inward pressure until a light pain can be felt in the jaw area.
- Hold for 5 seconds. Slowly release.
- Repeat at least 10 times.
- Use in conjunction with other *Instant Calm* techniques.

Cheekbone Press

This simple exercise works wonders in the relief of facial tension, eye strain and feelings of nervousness.

Press the tip of a forefinger against each cheekbone – directly below your eyes – with sufficient pressure to cause mild discomfort.

Maintain this pressure for 60 seconds, then release it.

Wait ten seconds and repeat. Do this up to five times.

CHEEKBONE PRESS

- Place the tip of the index finger against the cheekbones, directly below the eyes.
- Apply a direct inward pressure until a light pain can be felt.
- Hold for 60 seconds. Slowly release.
- Use in conjunction with Power Breathing techniques.

Front and Back Press

Acupressure is based on applying pressure to a series of energy pathways throughout the body known as meridians. Sometimes an acupressure treatment consists of nothing more than 'balancing' the energy in these pathways.

The Front and Back Press is a deceptively simple exercise that does just that. In doing so, it not only helps you to attain a state of calm, but also helps reduce tension around the head and neck areas.

In essence, it consists of one hand placed at the back of the neck just below the skull, with the other hand placed on the forehead. While neither hand should apply any significant pressure, they should initially feel like they are assuming control for the balance of your head and neck – taking all the effort from your neck muscles. When you can 'feel' that effect, let your arms relax while leaving both hands in place. For maximum effectiveness, right-handed people should place their right hands behind the neck, and left-handed people, vice versa.

If you then apply your Power Breathing technique, you will soon be overcome by a feeling of calm and peace. This is how it feels when your energy pathways are 'in balance'. (As an alternative, place one hand on your forehead and the other just below your navel.)

FRONT AND BACK PRESS

- Place your right hand at the back of the neck, at the base of the skull. (Left-handed people use left hand.) Place your left hand on your forehead. Exert effort with both hands to 'lift' the head from the body, thus removing the effort from your neck muscles. Then relax your arms.
- Commence Power Breathing techniques.
- Hold for 5 minutes.

Feng-chih

There are two significant acupressure points at the base of the skull – the occipital ridge – which, if pressed, not only relieve tension in the neck and shoulder area, but can induce a great feeling of calm.

Practitioners of shiatsu claim that less than a minute of consistent pressure to those points (known as *feng-chih* in Chinese medicine) can bring about total relaxation.

Another pressure point at the base of the skull is farther along – you will feel a slight ridge, just inside your sternocleidomastoid muscle (the muscle on the side of your neck behind the ear; it tightens when you turn your head to either side). Massaging this area with your thumbs for 30 seconds or so will provide relief.

How do you find them? Place your hands over the back of your skull so that your thumbs touch approximately at the level of the top of your spinal column. Feel for the base of your skull with your thumbs. Slide your thumbs outward (away from your vertebrae) along the skull bone. When your thumbs are about 5 centimetres (2 inches) apart, you will feel a ridge, a sensitive spot. Press on this, you will feel a dull pain (Figure 34).

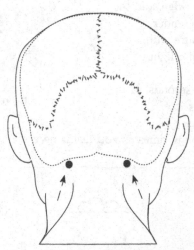

Figure 34

Now you are in the right area.

To ease a tension headache, and to produce a feeling of relaxation, simply apply an upward pressure with your thumbs against both of these points. When you are applying the correct amount, you will feel a little pain. If you are extremely tense, there could be quite a bit of discomfort. Persevere, and maintain the pressure for about 20 seconds longer if you can stand it. Then slowly ease off.

Repeat this exercise several times until your muscles relax.

(This is a technique you can either do yourself or have someone assist you.)

FENG-CHIH

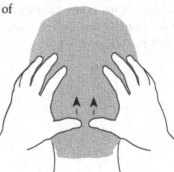

- With hands cradling the back of the skull, use thumbs to feel for the sensitive spot 2.5 centimetres (1 inch) or so out from the spinal column. You will feel the ridge, and the area may be tender.
- Apply pressure with thumbs until a light pain can be felt.
- Hold for 20 seconds, or longer if possible.

Figure 35

- Slowly release.
- Repeat as many times as you feel is necessary.

Heavenly Calm

Tsu-sanli

There is an acupressure point known as *tsu-sanli*, 'heavenly calm' in Chinese, which when massaged induces a state of relaxation.

To find it, sit with the left knee raised. Place the palm of your left hand on your kneecap (Figure 36). Immediately below the tip of your ring finger is the point you are concerned with.

Remove your hand from your knee.

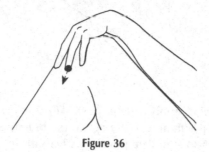

Figure 36

Using the nail – the tip of it – of your index finger, massage that point, *in a downward motion*, in short strokes about 2.5 centimetres (1 inch) in length. Do it rapidly, at about 100–120 strokes per minute.

The pressure applied should be heavy enough to stimulate the nerves beneath the skin, but not so heavy as to cause discomfort. Remember, though, the strokes must be in the same downward motion.

Then repeat the action on the right leg.

In most of the techniques that follow, a firm downward pressure with your finger can be substituted for the 'strokes' recommended.

NOTE: If pregnant, do not apply any acupressure techniques at points below the knee.

The stroking on both legs should take 5–10 minutes in total.

In severe cases of stress and anxiety, it is useful to adopt a programme of this and the following techniques, every second day.

Shao-chong

Another important acupressure point in the treatment of stress and anxiety is called *shao-chong*.

To find this point, place your left hand flat on a table, with your fingers spread. It is on the inside of the last joint of your little finger, just below the nail (Figure 37).

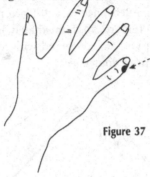

Figure 37

Using a fingernail, apply a series of strokes *from the inside out*, about 100–120 strokes per minute. Once again, the pressure applied should be heavy enough to stimulate the nerves beneath the skin, but not to cause discomfort. Repeat on the little finger of the right hand.

Jan-ku

The acupressure point in this treatment lies inside your foot.

To find it, go two finger-widths directly down from your inside ankle, then two finger-widths forward. You will feel a small indentation there. This is *jan-ku* (Figure 38).

Using the point of the finger-nail, apply a series of strokes

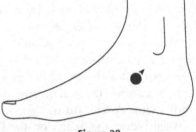

Figure 38

towards the ankle bone, about 100–120 strokes per minute. Once again, the pressure applied should be heavy enough to stimulate the nerves beneath the skin, but not to cause discomfort.

Continue this action on the same place on the right foot as well.

Chin-wei

The ideal is to use each of the preceding acupressure points (*tsu-sanli, shao-chong, jan-ku*) in sequence. *Chin-wei* is the final acupressure point in that series and is of no great use by itself. It is easy to find. It is at the lowest point of your breastbone – follow your ribs up and you can't miss it (Figure 39).

Using the point of the finger-nail, apply a series of strokes *upwards*, about 100–120 strokes per minute, with just enough pressure to stimulate the nerves beneath the skin, but not to cause discomfort.

In severe cases of stress and anxiety, it is useful to adopt a pro-gramme of this and the preceding techniques, every second day.

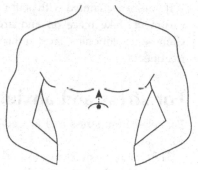

Figure 39

HEAVENLY CALM

- Find the acupressure point, as described, on the left leg, hand, ankle or breastbone.
- Using the point of your fingernail, make strokes about 2.5 centimetres (1 inch) in length – *in the direction indicated*. Do it rapidly, at about 100–120 strokes per minute.
- Repeat for the same place on the right leg, hand or ankle.
- Continue this action for 5–10 minutes, then sit somewhere quiet and allow the calm to envelop your body.
- For severe cases, begin a programme repeating these exercises every second day.

It's All in the Ear

In 1957, a Frenchman, Dr Paul Nogier, pioneered a new area in acupressure. He and his team mapped the individual parts of the body on the ear in a way similar to how the body is 'mapped' on the sole of the foot in reflexology.

If you're acquainted with acupuncture, you will be aware that many treatments take place on and around the ear – this is because the Chinese practitioners later utilised Dr Nogier's discoveries in their treatments.

For stress and anxiety

For relief from stress and anxiety, there are two important points on each ear.

The first of them is easy to find. It's at the lower front of the lobe of the right ear (Figure 40, a). Using the point of the fingernail, apply a series of strokes *upwards*, about 100–120 strokes per minute. Use just enough pressure to stimulate the nerves beneath the skin, but not to cause discomfort. Then find the corresponding spot on your left ear (b). This time, your strokes must go *downwards*.

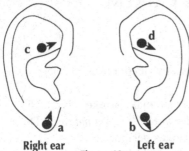

Right ear   **Left ear**

Figure 40

You'll need a friend or a mirror to find the second point in your right ear. There is a triangular-shaped hollow (c) near the top of your ear. Using the point of the fingernail, apply a series of strokes *forwards*, about 100–120 strokes per minute. Then find the corresponding spot on your left ear (d). This time, your strokes must go *backwards*.

After you have completed these exercises, sit somewhere quiet and allow the calm to envelop your body.

For tension and nervousness

There is another set of points around the ear that, stroked appropriately, can work wonders in the treatment of tension and nervousness.

The first point, on the right ear, is situated at the base of the piece of cartilage that joins the side of the face, just in front of the lowest hollow (Figure 41, a). Using the tip of the fingernail, apply a series of strokes *upwards*.

The second point on the right ear is situated at the lobe, but just below the lowest hollow (b). Apply a series of strokes *downwards*.

The third point is on the major ridge that sweeps down into the hollow of the ear (c). Apply a series of strokes *upwards and forwards*, along the natural line of the ridge.

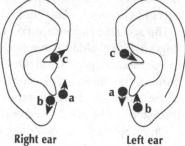

Then repeat these strokes on the left ear – but *reversing* the directions of the strokes.

After you have done the exercises, sit somewhere quiet and allow the calm to envelop your body.

Right ear   Left ear

Figure 41

IT'S ALL IN THE EAR

- Find the first acupressure point, as described, on your right ear lobe. Using the point of your fingernail, make strokes *in the direction indicated*. Do it rapidly, at about 100–120 strokes per minute.
- Repeat the action for the same place – *but in the direction indicated* – on the left ear.
- Continue each action for 5–10 minutes.
- Repeat for subsequent acupressure points, then sit somewhere quiet and allow the calm to envelop you.
- For cases of chronic stress, repeat these exercises every second day for a month.

Off the Top of the Head

Two other acupressure points for treating tension and nervousness are found at the top of the head.

The first of these, *pai-hui*, is at the centre of your skull, along an imaginary line drawn between your ears (Figure 42, a). Using the point of the fingernail, apply a series of strokes *forwards*, about 100–120 strokes per minute. Use just enough pressure to stimulate the nerves beneath the skin, but taking care not to cause discomfort.

The second acupressure point, *hou-ting*, is directly behind – three finger-widths behind – in a small indentation that is quite noticeable to the touch (Figure 42, b). Once again, apply a series of strokes *forwards*, in the direction of your face.

Use both of these exercises in conjunction with the *chin-wei* (breastbone – Figure 39) exercise.

On completion, rest quietly until you feel a sense of calm take over.

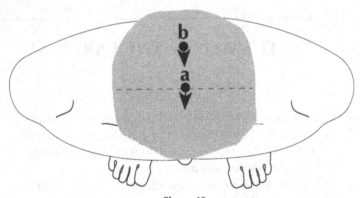

Figure 42

OFF THE TOP OF THE HEAD

- Find the first acupressure point (a) at the crown of the head, at the point midway between your ears.
- Using the point of your fingernail, make strokes *forwards*. Do this rapidly, at about 100–120 strokes per minute. Continue this action for 5 minutes.
- Find the second acupressure point (b) at an indentation about three finger-widths behind that.
- Using the point of your fingernail, make strokes *forwards*. Do this rapidly, at about 100–120 strokes per minute. Continue the action for 5 minutes.
- Follow with the *chin-wei* exercise from page 160–1.
- On completion, rest quietly until you feel a sense of calm take over.

The Calm Wrist

One of the most important acupressure points for the treatment of anxiety is located in the centre of your wrist, in a line from your middle finger, about two thumb-widths from the bottom of your palm (Figure 43a). This is known as *nei-kuan*.

You can treat this in one of two ways – either by applying a series of strokes *forwards* with the point of the fingernail (about 100–120 strokes per minute), or by pressing on it with the thumb of your other hand.

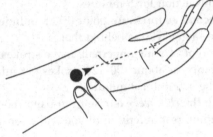

Figure 43a

(You can use this latter technique – simply pressing instead of massaging – on many of the other acupressure points mentioned in this book.)

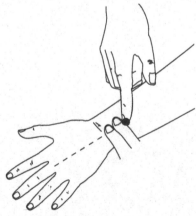

Figure 43b

As you press against the point, take a deep, diaphragmatic breath, being careful not to let your shoulders rise. Then follow it with a long, slow exhalation.

This is a most effective technique. You should start to feel relief almost immediately after applying it.

An alternative acupressure point is on the upper side of your wrist, directly up from your middle finger, about two thumb-widths above the crease of your wrist (Figure 43b). It is virtually above the *nei-kuan* point mentioned above.

Applying a strong, downward pressure with your forefinger, thumb or knuckle, massage here in a counter-clockwise direction for 20 seconds.

Repeat this process on the other wrist, and continue until you find relief.

THE CALM WRIST

- Find acupressure point (a) at the centre of your wrist, about two thumb-widths back from the bottom of your palm, or (b) on the upper side of your wrist about two thumb-widths from the crease.
- Using the thumb (forefinger or knuckle) of your other hand, press firmly on this point.
- Take a deep, diaphragmatic breath, then follow with a long, slow exhalation.
- Massage the point for 20–30 seconds. In the case of point (a) ensure you massage *forwards*. With point (b), massage in a *counter-clockwise* direction.
- Repeat with other wrist. Continue the process until you find relief.

Very Calm Wrist

There is an even more potent acupressure point on your wrist than either of the two just covered. It is at the crease of your inner wrist, in a line directly from your little finger (Figure 44).

When you have isolated the point, apply a strong, downward pressure – with your forefinger, thumb or knuckle – and massage in a counter-clockwise direction for 20 seconds. Repeat this process on the other wrist, and continue until relief is at hand.

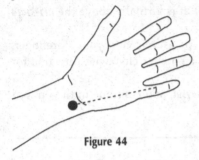

Figure 44

Reserve this point for extreme cases. In these events, you should massage it, on both wrists, only once. Then go on to any of the other treatments in this book.

VERY CALM WRIST

(Use only in extreme cases)

- Find the acupressure point at the bottom of your palm, directly back from your little finger.
- Using the thumb, forefinger or knuckle of your other hand, press firmly on this point.
- Take a deep, diaphragmatic breath, then follow with a long, slow exhalation.
- Massage the point for 20 seconds.
- Repeat with other wrist.
- If relief is not complete, continue with any of the other techniques in this book.

Calm Hands

Here's a simple technique you can access anywhere, any time, for a fast and effective relaxation. However, it is not suitable for pregnant women.

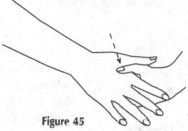

Figure 45

There's an acupressure point at the top of your hand in the 'V' where the bones of your thumb and forefinger meet. You will feel it distinctly – not only because it is obvious to the touch, but because it's also a sensitive spot when you press on it. Applying pressure to this point has a distinct calming effect on the body, and a soothing effect on the emotions.

To apply the pressure, pinch with your thumb and forefinger of the other hand until it hurts.

CALM HANDS

- Find the sensitive acupressure point at top of your hand near the bones from the thumb and forefinger meet.
- Using the thumb and forefinger of your other hand, squeeze firmly on this point.
- Maintaining the pressure, take a deep Power Breath, then follow with a long, slow exhalation.
- Continue Power Breathing for 5 breaths.
- Repeat with other hand.

More Calm Points

Following are a number of other acupressure points which, used correctly, are simple and effective ways of relieving a variety of conditions that relate to stress, tension and anxiety.

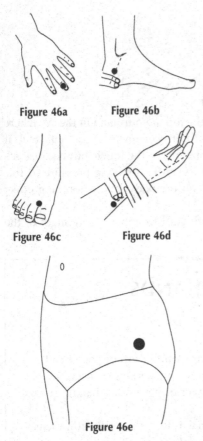

Figure 46a

Figure 46b

Figure 46c

Figure 46d

Figure 46e

There are many more, of course, than the four covered here. However these have been chosen for two reasons: you can access them yourself and they're relatively easy to find, even for a novice.

Each of these points is treated by a firm downwards pressure with the forefinger or thumb, massaged in a clockwise direction for 20 seconds. Continue until you find relief.

The first point is on the middle finger, between the nail and the first joint, slightly on the thumb-side of centre (Figure 46a). As you press against the point, take a deep Power Breath, followed by a long, slow exhalation.

The second point is on the inside of your foot. If you draw an imaginary line from the middle of your ankle to the tip of your heel, you will find the point two thumb-widths from the heel (Figure 46b).

Applying pressure to this point reduces tension and feelings of anxiety. (Pregnant women should avoid this.)

The third point is at the top of your foot, in the indentation between your big and second toes (Figure 46c).

As you press against the point, take a deep, diaphragmatic breath, being careful not to let your shoulders rise. Then follow it with a long, slow exhalation. (Again, this is not a point suitable for pregnant women.)

The fourth point is on the side of your forearm, in a line directly back from the side of your little finger, the width of four fingers and two thumbs from the crease of your wrist (Figure 46d). You will feel the indentation and its sensitivity. Massage this point while you apply your Power Breathing techniques.

The last point is easily found in the hollow of your hip. You may need to use a mirror to find it, but it is an obvious point – a small indentation at the ball joint of the hip (Figure 46e) which is most notice-able when your squeeze your buttocks together.

When you find this point, relax the muscles in your buttocks and use your Power Breathing as you apply pressure.

Pause after each pressure application, using your Power Breathing technique as you wait for the sense of calm to overtake you.

Do-it-yourself Massage (A)

Massage is not generally considered a therapy you can apply on yourself. There are, however, a couple of major exceptions. What follows is a series of massage strokes that, *in combination*, will have a fairly imme-diate soothing effect in stressful situations.

Perform these massage exercises with essential oils from page 245 and the results will be doubly powerful.

They are derived from shiatsu (which would normally involve pres-sures rather than strokes) and are some of the easiest, most pleasurable and natural-feeling exercises in this book.

The first takes place around the eye sockets (Figure 47a). The massage action is conducted with the thumb, index and middle finger of each hand, kneading *outwards* in a circular motion.

Do this ten times.

Then reverse the kneading action *inwards*, also ten times.

The second action involves an acupressure point that has a powerful influence on the way you feel – massaging this point is said to relieve depression as well as feelings of pressure. Indeed, it is a point that you instinctively reach for when you're under pressure.

It's the point at your temples, the *tae yang* (Figure 47b).

Using the tips of the middle finger of each hand massage *forwards*, in a circular motion, ten times. Then massage *backwards*, also in a circular motion, ten times.

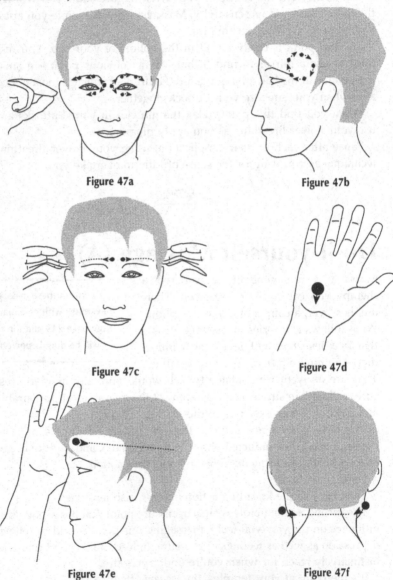

Figure 47a

Figure 47b

Figure 47c

Figure 47d

Figure 47e

Figure 47f

The next exercise is also performed with the tips of the middle fingers.

From a point between the eyebrows, draw a straight line towards the temples, then continue towards the back of the head (Figure 47c). Do this twenty times.

The fourth exercise in this sequence utilises not the fingertips, but the heels of your palms (Figure 47d). Applying a reasonable pressure to either side of your head starting at your forehead – just below your hairline – slide your hands right around your head until your hands meet at the back (Figure 47e). Do this thirty times.

The final exercise in this series takes place at the back of the neck. Using the thumb and fingers of your right hand, apply pressure at the base of your skull, about three finger-widths in from your ears (Figure 47f). Then, in a fluid, squeezing motion, slide your fingers in towards the base of the neck.

Do this ten times.

After you have completed this series of exercises, sit quietly for 10 minutes concentrating on your Power Breathing, and allow the feeling of calm to filter through your body.

Do-it-yourself Massage (B)

This series of exercises differs from those preceding in that they are more relaxed and sensuous in their application. Their similarity is that they concentrate on the head and face areas, where stress concentrates most of all.

Before you begin, though, make a commitment to yourself to enjoy the experience you are about to embark on. That commitment alone is an effective path to relaxation.

The first of these exercises is simply a head massage (Figure 48a). Do this in whichever way feels best to you – a vigorous 'shampoo-rub' technique, or a slow, firm pressure from spread fingers. Combine both, if you like.

Do this for 60 seconds, or longer if you prefer.

The rest of these exercises concentrate on the facial areas.

First, cover your eyes with the palms of your hands allowing your

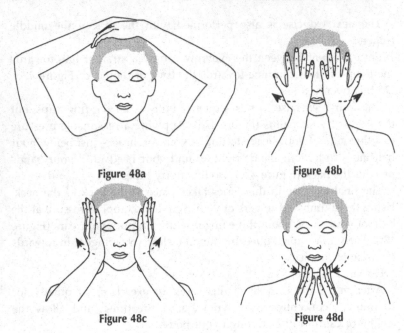

Figure 48a

Figure 48b

Figure 48c

Figure 48d

nose to peek through (Figure 48b). While Power Breathing, apply a firm pressure to your face so the heels of your palms press just beneath your cheekbones. Hold this position for 10 seconds or so, then slowly slide your hands around your face, lightly dragging your skin and facial muscles as you do so.

When your hands reach the side of your face, gently slide them up so you can feel your skin and facial muscles being pulled upwards in a 'face lift' action (Figure 48c). Do this as slowly as you can.

Maintain your Power Breathing all this while, and you will begin to feel relief as your facial muscles relax.

When you can feel these muscles relax, *softly* run your fingertips – barely caressing your skin – down your cheeks, beneath your chin, until they slowly lose contact with your skin (Figure 48d).

You skin should be lightly tingling at this stage.

Repeat this sequence as many times as you like – ensuring that you maintain your Power Breathing as you do so.

On completion, sit somewhere quiet for 10 minutes and luxuriate in the feeling of calm that surrounds you.

Calm Nose Job

As we have already seen, there are a number of important stress-relieving acupressure points around the eye and nose area. Some of these points may be more difficult to find than others but, because they usually have the most pronounced and immediate effects, the results will be well worth the initial search.

Around the area of the eye socket are three vital points. Although the illustration (Figure 49) shows approximately where they are, only experimentation will reveal their precise location.

These points are usually quite sensitive. If you are tense, your search will be made easier because they will be more sensitive than usual. Even when you are relaxed, a light application of pressure should be all it takes to identify them.

The first point (a) is easiest to find. It is where the eyebrow bone meets the bridge of the nose. Press gently against the eyebrow bone and you will feel it.

The second point (b) is also under the eyebrow bone, but directly up from the iris. It is on the *inside* edge of a small indentation you will be able to feel with your thumb. (If you wear contact lenses, be sure to remove them before applying pressure to this point.)

The third point (c) is directly beneath or behind (b), further *back* into the eye socket. If you place your fingernail against (b), pressing in gently until your finger presses against the eyeball, you will be able to feel the point directly above. Naturally areas (b) and (c) should be treated gently.

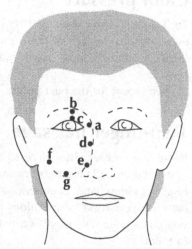

Figure 49

Points (d) and (e) run alongside the nose. The upper point (d) is in a small groove just below where the eye socket touches the nose. The lower point (e) rests in the indentation between the nostril and the cheek bone.

The points (f) and (g) are removed from the general nose area. The upper point (f) is easiest found when you open your mouth wide; it is on the outer edge of your jaw muscle, just below the cheekbone. It's a sensitive point, you won't miss it.

The lowest point, (g), is below your cheekbone, just above the upper level of your teeth. Once again, it is a sensitive point so should be easily found.

Whether you choose to use pressure (preferable) or the two-finger massage, it is important to remember two things.

a   This series of exercises is meant to be soothing – so take your time and enjoy the sensuousness of the experience; remember your Power Breathing as you perform them.
b   On completion, sit quietly for 10 minutes and wait for a sense of calm to envelop you.

Calm pressure

To find relief from stress and tension, all you have to do is apply an even pressure to each of these points (lightly in the eye socket area, firmly around the nose area) and maintain for 10 seconds. Release slowly.

Then repeat for the next point.

Two-finger massage

Possibly an easier alternative to applying pressure to each of these points individually is a two-finger massage. Using the thumb and fore-finger of either hand, commence a long fluid massage stroke from the *outside* the eye socket, down along the nose, around the cheekbone until you reach point (f) – there is a natural course all the way that is easy to follow.

Then reverse the action.

Do this thirty times.

Foot Relaxations

The exercises that follow are an ideal way to begin any relaxation session. Whether you choose to follow them with other reflexology exercises or not, you will find them soothing and relaxing in their own right. Better still, these are exercises you can perform yourself.

There are five of them in the series.

Before you begin, find a quiet, restful place and take a minute or so to prepare. First soak your feet or clean them with a warm wet towel, then rub in a little moisturiser, body cream or, best of all, a relaxing combination of essential oils.

Perform all of the exercises on one foot before moving to the other.

FOOT RELAXATIONS

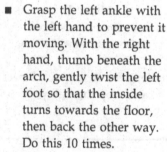

- Grasp the left ankle with the left hand to prevent it moving. With the right hand, thumb beneath the arch, gently twist the left foot so that the inside turns towards the floor, then back the other way. Do this 10 times.
- Massage each toe individually, then stretch (a). Rotate each toe one way, then back (b). Perform each movement 10 times.

continued on page 178

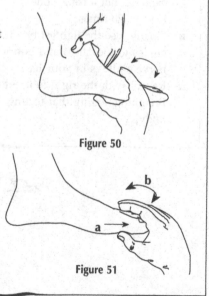

Figure 50

Figure 51

- Firmly hold the top of your foot – just behind the toes – with your left hand. Form a fist with your right hand and press up from beneath. Now alternate pressing up with your right fist (a), then squeezing with your left hand (b). Do this 10 times.

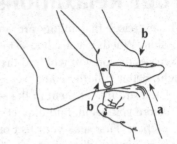

Figure 52

- Make sure the ankle is loose and relaxed. With a hand on either side of the foot, lightly toss it from one side to the other. This should be a stimulating exercise, not a rough one. Do this 20 times.

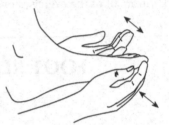

Figure 53

- Finally, use the lightest brush of your fingertips – from ankles to toes, tops and bottoms of feet – to sensitise the nerve endings in your feet.
- Repeat with the right foot. Sit quietly for 10 minutes, Power Breathing, letting that feeling of calm seep through your body.

20

THIRD PARTY PRESSURES

Whereas most of the relaxation techniques featured so far have been designed to be performed by yourself, some of the more powerful of them require a third party to assist.

This is a time-proven way of sharing your stress or anxiety. But there is yet another, more relaxing, aspect: when someone else

The involvement of another person is a time-proven way of sharing your stress or anxiety; in many cases, simply the presence of another adds to the calming effect.

assists, you can just sit back and take it easy while they assume all the responsibility and apply all the effort.

The following exercises require the assistance of a willing associate. And, once again, they are made all the more powerful if performed with calming essential oils.

Deep Face Massage

This soothing pair of exercises requires only a modicum of sensitivity and skill from the massager.

They are designed to do two things: to provide a sensation of physical warmth and comfort to the recipient, and to reduce the tensions that accumulate in the large muscles of the face. Also, as we have seen with earlier techniques, these exercises stimulate many of the important acupressure points found in this area.

The following instructions are for the person applying the treatment.

Begin by resting the palm of the hand on each side of the face (Figure 54a) – the bottom of the palms covering the lips, and the fingertips covering the eyes. Leave your hands there, unmoving, until you can feel the subject's body heat. Wait another 30 seconds.

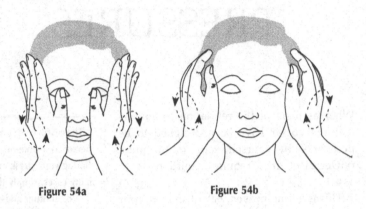

Figure 54a   **Figure 54b**

With a modest downward pressure, and an *outward* circular motion, slowly massage the area that your hands cover. Do this *without lifting them from the facial surface.*

Maintain this movement for whatever length of time you sense is necessary – it will be at least 2 minutes.

The second exercise employs a similar technique. This time the hands are placed over each temple with the thumbs resting against the ears (Figure 54b).

Ensuring that you massage beneath the skin, with your hands not leaving the facial surface, begin a circular motion towards the back of the head. Maintain this movement for a minimum of 2 minutes.

Although brief, those few minutes of massage will dissolve most tensions that concentrate in a tense person's face. These actions alone should induce a powerful feeling of calm. If, however, tension persists, simply repeat the exercise or combine it with the following.

Four-point Facial Massage

At first glance, the following exercises may seem complicated. This is an illusion. Indeed, perform them only once and you will be surprised at how natural and intuitive they are. Moreover, each of the exercises in this group is linked – one leads naturally to the next. Be aware of this continuity, and the massage will become second nature to you.

Ensure your subject is reclining comfortably, breathing deeply, eyes closed.

Begin with your right hand covering his or her face, palm on forehead, barely touching the skin (Figure 55a). Feel the body heat being drawn into the palm of your hand. With a forefinger and ring finger

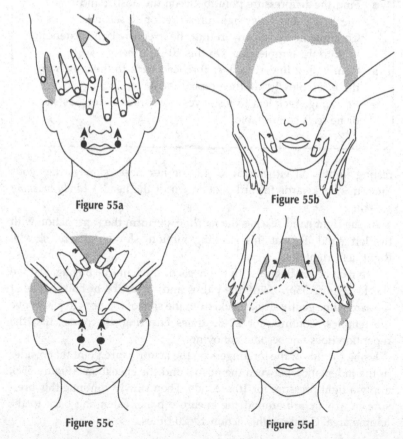

Figure 55a

Figure 55b

Figure 55c

Figure 55d

FOUR-POINT FACIAL MASSAGE

- Lightly cover his or her face with your right hand. Slowly drag fingertips towards the crown. As the right hand reaches the hairline, do the same with the left hand. Repeat this slow, stroking motion.
- With palms and fingertips of both hands, gently stroke back from the neck to above the temples. Continue 20–30 times.
- Find the acupressure point between the nostril and cheekbone and apply light pressure for 10 seconds. Continue in a wide arc around the eyebrow bone, extending back to the temple area. Do this 10–20 times.
- Gently drag fingertips over forehead back to the crown of the head. Slowly lift, then repeat the action.
- Encourage recipient to rest, eyes closed, for as long as she or he feels comfortable.

resting lightly on either side of his or her nose, slowly drag your fingertips backwards towards the crown of the head – *barely touching the skin*.

As the right hand reaches the hairline, perform the same action with the left hand. Repeat this stroking motion, slowly, slowly, slowly. Right, left, right, left.

The next action begins with the heels of the hand resting against the cheeks (Figure 55b). Using the palms and fingertips of both hands at the same time gently stroke back, from the side of the neck to just above the temples. Continue for 20–30 times ensuring, of course, that the repetition does not become annoying.

Using the tips of the forefingers on the acupressure point that resides in the indentation between the nostril and the cheekbone (Figure 55c), apply a light pressure for 10 seconds. Then slowly continue this pressure in a wide arc around the eyebrow bone, extending back to the temple area. Continue this action 10–20 times.

The last action in this sequence begins in the temple area (Figure 55d). It should be considered the culmination of the exercise sequence and be performed with an intuitive balance between firmness and lightness of touch – in other words, *you* make the choice at the time of massage.

With the fingertips spread lightly against around the temple area, gently draw them over the forehead, up to the hairline, back to the crown of the head. Then slowly lift them and repeat the action.

Remember, though, that this is the finale of the treatment – even though you may repeat the sequence several times – and should be conducted *with a progressively lighter and slower touch.*

After you have completed these exercises, withdraw your hands and encourage your subject to rest, eyes closed, for as long as she or he feels comfortable.

Beauty Facial Massage

Probably the leading exponents of the facial massage are the modern beauty salons. Following is a series of massage techniques loosely based on the treatments given in these salons.

These techniques are most effective when performed with calming essential oils or facial lotions. If using skin-care lotions be sure to choose thin, soothing types – as opposed to thick or sticky creams and astringents.

Figure 56 is a map of the most calming massage patterns. When applying them, slowly slide the fingers along the route shown as a dotted line, pausing and applying a reasonably firm downward pressure at the points indicated.

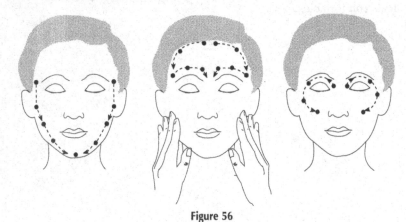

Figure 56

The first is a natural-flowing line from temple to the top of the cheekbone, to the indentation behind the cheekbone, to the muscle at the corner of the jawbone, to the edge of the chin, through to the point of the chin.

The second covers the forehead area. It begins at the highest central point of the forehead and traces a line to the temples, around the eyebrows, coming to rest at the acupressure point at the corner of each eyebrow. At each of these points, pause a few seconds, applying a moderate pressure.

The third sequence involves a number of the acupressure points we covered in an earlier technique, the Calm Nose Job (page 175).

It begins at the point where the eyebrow bone meets the bridge of the nose, continues to the indentation at the highest point of the eyebrow bone, to the outer point of the eyebrow socket, to the temple area, to the outer edge of your jaw muscle, to the indentation between the nostril and the cheekbone. Describe a wide arc around these areas, pausing and applying light pressure at each of the points.

Take as long as you can in performing these massages. Linger over them. Put as much tenderness and feeling into them as you can. The results will be well worth your effort – you will have worked wonders in removing the stress from another person.

When complete, urge your subject to lie back and relax for 10 minutes or so.

Lower Back Massage

For reasons we have already outlined, many sufferers of stress find that it makes its presence most felt in the lower back. Often, even those who are unaware of pain in this area are surprised to discover how much pent-up discomfort there is – when the area is massaged.

> You can make your own massage oil by adding a few drops of calming essential oils (see page 245) to a bland carrier oil such as sweet almond or apricot kernel.

The following massage technique is both basic and intuitive; you have probably used something similar to it at some time or another yourself. What makes it attractive, though, is how easy it is to perform. In fact, considering the minimal level of skill or effort that it requires, lower back massage can be quite astounding in the relief it affords.

To begin with, lower the lights and consider playing relaxing 'ambience' music. Have your subject lie on his or her stomach, unclothed from the upper buttocks to the middle of the back.

Spread a massage oil or body lotion over the area to be massaged. (Be sure to warm the oil first, to a little above room temperature; a shock of *cold* oil does not lend itself to helping someone feel calm.) Then follow the detailed instructions that follow.

LOWER BACK MASSAGE

■ Start with a light, almost superficial stroking of the lower back towards the shoulders. Continue this for as long as it takes to relax your subject.

■ Then, with one of your hands pressing on the other, apply a deep massage action to the muscles of the buttocks. This will be a heavy kneading action with the

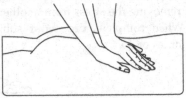

Figure 57a

flat of your hand – you will need to press fairly heavily to have the desired effect, though be careful not to cause too much discomfort. Do this at least 5 times on either side.

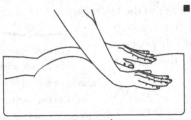

Figure 57b

■ Moving up to the lumbar muscles in the small of the back, begin to massage from the top of the buttocks to the waist. When you have completed both massage actions – and this will probably take several minutes – either continue further up the back to the shoulder area, or recommence the light, almost superficial stroking that you began with.

■ Continue for as long as you feel necessary, taking care not to over-work the muscles. When you sense your subject is in a state of deep relaxation, you can discontinue these massage actions, and encourage him or her to lie there, luxuriating in the peace of the moment.

Neck and Shoulder Massage

The neck and shoulder area is the most noticeable place in the body for stress-related discomfort to concentrate.

Even the most unskilled massage in this area will provide an immediate relief. At the very minimum, the process will be both soothing and pleasurable.

Lower the lights, ensure the room is warm and, if you choose, turn on relaxing ambience music. Begin with your subject on his or her stomach, unclothed from the waist up. Spread warm massage oil or body lotion over the back and shoulders, then follow the instructions in the box.

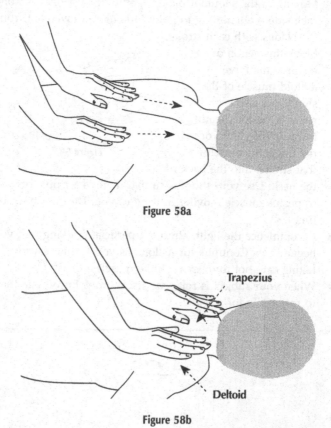

Figure 58a

Trapezius

Deltoid

Figure 58b

NECK AND SHOULDER MASSAGE

- Start with a light, almost superficial stroking of the shoulder blade area until your subject is relaxed.
- With a hand on either side of the spine, apply a deep massage action from the middle of the back towards the shoulders. Do this 10 times, extending the length of stroke each time.
- Moving to the shoulder blades, apply deep strokes – 5 on each side – attempting to get a little more movement from the blades with each stroke.
- Move this action out towards the large deltoid muscle of the shoulders. Use a rounded action, heading towards the centre of the trapezius muscles that stretch into the back of the neck. Use your thumbs so that there is a ripple of trapezius muscle moving in front of you. Do this about 10 times.

Figure 59

- Recommence the light, almost superficial stroking that you began with. Continue for as long as you feel necessary, taking care not to over-work the muscles.
- When your subject is relaxed, discontinue. Encourage them to rest easily for a while.

Simple Reflexology

According to reflexology theory, the feet are mini-maps of the body and its organs. By applying pressures to specific areas of the foot, a reflexologist strives to unblock energy channels and thus relieve specific ailments or discomforts in other parts of the body. In many ways, it is like the system of pressure points used in acupressure and shiatsu massage.

Like many other 'alternative' therapies, reflexology sometimes attracts a degree of scepticism. I am regularly asked whether I subscribe to the claims attributed to it. Not all of them. However, I am certain that, within the context of *Instant Calm*, a reflexology treatment will make most people feel dramatically more relaxed.

The following exercises are simple and easy to follow. But, first, it is worthwhile examining the areas of your subject's feet that influence the way he or she copes with stress.

In a quiet, restful place, perform the following exercises on one foot before progressing to the other.

First, grasp the ankle with one hand and shake it gently from side to side until the foot is relaxed (Figure 60a). As a warm up, massage each toe individually, then stretch – rotating each of them one way, then back (Figure 60b).

Next, supporting the top of the foot with one hand, use the thumb

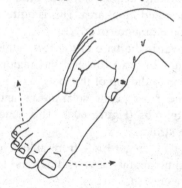

Figure 60a

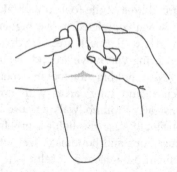

Figure 60b

Next, supporting the top of the foot with one hand, use the thumb to work around the 'solar plexus' area (Figure 60c). Simply bend the thumb at the first joint in a series of tiny, stepped, 'walking' movements. Endeavour to do this as smoothly, with as even a pressure as possible. Then, if you can do it comfortably, rotate the foot from one side to the other, pivoting on your thumb.

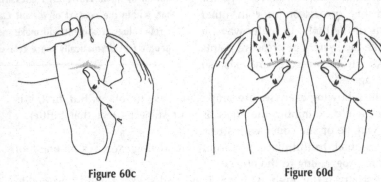

Figure 60c   **Figure 60d**

Work this area for a minute or longer, until you feel your subject slip into a deep state of relaxation.

Now, with your subject relaxed, you are ready to progress to other parts of the body. Using the same 'walking' action with your thumbs, move higher up the foot into the 'chest and lung' area. This is quite a broad area of the foot so will take some time to cover.

When completed, move higher towards the base of the toes – this relates to the neck area – and continue to 'walk' around this region, ensuring you move around the big toe to the top of the foot.

Next, holding one foot in either hand, massage the 'solar plexus' and 'chest and lung' areas with your thumbs (Figure 60d). This time, instead of thumb 'walking', use long strokes.

Finally, use the lightest brush of your fingertips – from ankles to toes, tops and bottoms of feet – to stimulate the nerve endings and to enhance the feeling of calm you have created.

REFLEXOLOGY AREAS

- On top of the foot, across the top of the big toe, is the area that relates to the region around the neck's C7 vertebra – where so much tension seems to accumulate.
- On the sole of the foot, the band across the end of the toes relates to the head, while the band across the bottom of the toes relates to the neck – both areas where the negative effects of stress are pronounced.

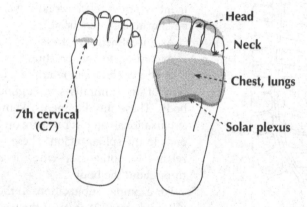

- The large area at the ball of the foot relates to the chest and lungs, while the indentation just below it relates to the solar plexus and stomach – also areas aggravated by the effects of stress and tension.

Chiropractic

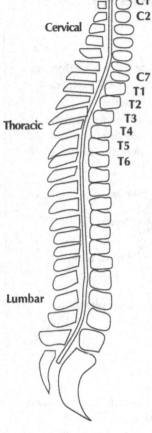

C1
C2
Cervical

C7
T1
T2
T3
Thoracic
T4
T5
T6

Lumbar

Figure 61

As there is little likelihood of an untrained person performing chiropractic treatments, there is no need to cover what follows in great detail. It may be beneficial, however, if I outline some of the positive benefits of chiropractic as a treatment for stress-related conditions.

Contrary to common belief, chiropractic has uses over and above the traditional stiff back or neck. As a preventative healing art, and as a treatment for stress-related conditions, it can be enormously beneficial.

As a treatment for stress?

According to the practitioners, misaligned vertebrae can interfere with the flow of nerve impulses throughout the body. These misalignments, known as subluxations, can put pressure on nerve ends in the spinal region. These nerves relate to other specific locations throughout the body.

For example, subluxations in the *atlas* (C1) and *axis* (C2) areas of the neck can cause problems with the *greater occipital nerve*. This, in turn, can cause headache, feelings of anxiety and tension – in other words, 'stressful' feelings.

Similarly, subluxations in the upper *thoracic* area of the spine (T1– T5) can cause pain or feelings of tightness in the chest – feelings that are commonly described as 'stressful'. Subluxations in T6 can cause tension and discomfort in the stomach area – the feeling associated with stress, once again.

Conversely, tight muscles around the head, neck and lower back regions – all of which can be aggravated by stress – can lead to subluxations in nearby vertebrae. In turn, these subluxations can lead to stressful feelings in the areas where the related nerve ends surface. It can be a vicious cycle.

A chiropractor can interrupt this cycle.

Devotees insist that chiropractic treatment of those subluxations – by a qualified practitioner, of course – usually provides instant relief from the feelings of stress that are associated with them.

I am one such devotee.

21

CALM DEVICES

It is the dream of every stressed person to discover a simple device that will instantly induce a state of calm – without commitment, without effort.

If the stressed person exhibits Type A personality characteristics, that dream becomes even more desirable.

But is this wishful thinking of the most extreme kind? If such devices existed, wouldn't Paul Wilson be marketing them rather than spending years researching a book on the topic?

I will confess that I've searched long and hard for the miracle solution.

What follows are a few of the discoveries I've turned up. While they do rely on physical devices for their effect, they also require a level of effort and commitment on your part.

And, even if some of them aren't quite as convenient, immediate, or as portable as other techniques in this book, they do work.

Moreover, some of them are quite extraordinary in what they can achieve.

Finger Bindings

One of the cornerstone concepts of zone therapy (see page 152) is the idea of the body being divided into ten separate electromagnetic fields, or zones. The organs, glands and nerves in each of these zones can be accessed via a corresponding part of the hand or foot.

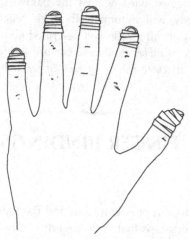

Figure 62

For example, the thumb of the right hand relates to the pituitary, pineal and thyroid glands, the throat, pancreas, bladder and so on. According to the principles of zone therapy, if you massage the thumb you stimulate all of those organs. Similarly, if you massage the fore-finger you stimulate a different group of organs.

Practitioners of zone therapy apply a daily massage to all fingers of each hand – thus treating and relaxing the entire body in a single session.

An alternative to this is a rather curious, but apparently effective, practice called Finger Bindings.

It requires no special skills and little effort. All you have to do is wrap ordinary rubber bands around the tops of the thumb and each finger (Figure 62). Wrap them tightly until your fingertips turn blue. (Naturally you should discontinue this if they become too uncomfortable.) With these bands in place, clench your hand tightly for 3 minutes.

Then relax.

Repeat with the other hand – and toes, if you choose.

Remove your Finger Bindings, wait 5 minutes, then repeat the exercise. If you can manage this daily, it works wonders for relaxing the nervous system.

(You may recognise the action I have just described. It is similar to the body's usual response to stress or tension – tightly clasped hands, with fingertips pressed hard against the palms. In stressful circumstances, your body will automatically seek relief by employing a clenching and unclenching action as described above.)

As an alternative to rubber bands you can use spring-loaded clothes pegs which you simply attach to the tip of each finger and leave in place for 5 minutes or more.

FINGER BINDINGS

- Wrap ordinary rubber bands around the tops of the thumb and each finger, so that your fingertips turn blue.
- Clench your hand tightly for 3 minutes. Then relax.
- Repeat with the other hand – and toes, if you choose.
- Remove your Finger Bindings, wait 5 minutes, then repeat the exercise.
- Sit somewhere quiet for 10 minutes, Power Breathing, and allow the feeling of calm to envelop you.
- If you can manage this daily, it works wonders for relaxing the nervous system.

Comb Therapy

Another curious relaxation technique employed in zone therapy dupli-
cates the intense stroking action of massage with the stroke of an aluminium, or possibly even a plastic, comb.

Employing a series of *upwards* motions,
stroke the comb over the fingers and
fingertips – both on top of and beneath the
hands. Extend these strokes up the wrists,
arms, all the way up to the shoulders.

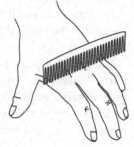

Repeat this action on the feet as well.

This pleasant-feeling exercise may be
extended as long as you desire, and is particularly useful for feelings of nervousness,
fatigue and poor circulation.

Figure 63

If you couple Comb Therapy with a 3-minute pressure on the tongue
(use the handle of your toothbrush or a spoon), the benefits are even
more pronounced.

COMB THERAPY

- Take an ordinary aluminium hair comb, and employ a
  series of upward strokes over fingers and fingertips.
- Extend these up the wrists, arms, all the way to the
  shoulders.
- Repeat action on the other hand. Do it on the feet as well.
- Couple this with a 3-minute pressure on the top of the
  tongue (an acupressure point) with the handle of a
  toothbrush or a spoon.
- Sit somewhere quiet for 10 minutes, Power Breathing, and
  allow the feeling of calm to envelop you.

The Balls of your Feet

One of the more innovative stress-relief devices I've come across is one you may already have in your house.

It's a tennis ball. An ordinary tennis ball.

No, you don't use it like one of those 'stress balls' (squishy balls you squeeze in the hand) that sell in executive shops. You roll it under your foot.

Utilising the principles of reflexology we touched upon in Third Party Pressures on page 191, this technique accesses the many pressure points (nerve endings) that exist in the feet. Stimulating these nerve endings – by applying pressure in the appropriate places – releases tension throughout much of the body, not just in the feet and leg areas.

THE BALLS OF YOUR FEET

- Place an ordinary tennis ball beneath the arch of your bare foot.
- Using a comfortable downward pressure, move your foot forwards and backwards – so that the ball moves from the toes to the heel.

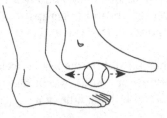

- Do this for 2 minutes on your left foot, then 2 minutes on your right.
- Repeat as necessary. Combine it with Power Breathing exercises.

Figure 64

The Balls of your Neck

This is a simple, but ingenious, way of finding relief from the tensions that build up in your back, neck and cranium muscles. It is a more colourful alternative to the rolled towel method covered earlier in the Feet Up Technique and, for some, is simpler than the Feng-chih acupressure also covered earlier.

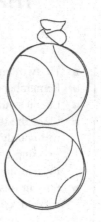

The device at the centre of this technique is one you can manufacture with the utmost ease. Simply stick two tennis balls in a sock and tie a knot in it.

That's it?

With this trusty device at your disposal, tension and tension headache are easily treated, and relaxation is close at hand.

Simply lie on the floor with your feet up, with your neck nestled in between those balls – the pressure they exert is ideal for releasing the most fierce tensions. Why? Because they work directly on the *feng-chih* acupressure points at the base of your skull, and they also apply a relieving pressure on the taut sternocleidomastoid muscles towards the side of your neck.

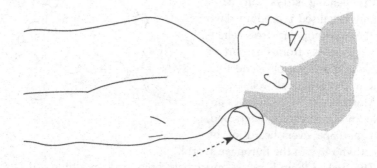

Figure 65

THE BALLS OF YOUR NECK

- Tie two tennis balls tightly in a sock.
- Remember the Conditions of Calm.
- Lie on your back on the floor, with your feet on a chair.
- Place the tennis balls behind your upper neck, so that they rest snugly against the skull ridge. The pressure of the balls pressing against the base of your skull will force your taut muscles to relax. If you feel dizzy, sit up.
- Stay in this position for at least 10–20 minutes. When relaxed, employ other techniques from this book.

Worry Beads

In the Middle East, overcoming or preventing stress can be a highly ritualised procedure. Two of the most popular stress-relieving techniques from this part of the world are not only effective, but are intriguing as well.

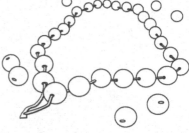

Moreover, these techniques are seldom appreciated, understood, nor perhaps even heard of by most who live in the European world.

The first of them is not so much a technique as an attitude. It is a perspective on time that works wonders in the elimination of (or, more correctly, in the avoidance of) anxiety.

Where most Europeans 'view' time as something stretching out before them – sequentially, where each step follows the one before it, and where each task sits waiting ahead of the next (Figure 66a) – many in the Middle East 'view' it in a more immediate sense.

To apply a visual perspective: in the Middle Eastern concept, time is 'seen' as something crossing their paths (Figure 66b), rather than something that stretches before them. Even though the difference is subtle, this simple variation in perspective makes it possible to ignore the future and to live in the present; and if you can ignore the future, you can avoid *all* anxieties and anxious conditions. Conversely, the sequential future-oriented concept of time that most Europeans use encourages anxiety – because anxiety always relates to the future.

(While some psychotherapists utilise variations on this concept in treating stressed individuals, it is not a concept easily adopted by Europeans. I have included it here as a matter of interest only.)

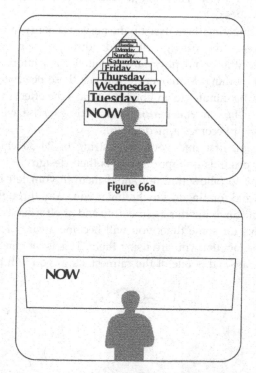

Figure 66a

Figure 66b

The second technique utilised by some Middle Eastern people is one we can all relate to – even if we do not understand the underlying principle of its use.

It is the technique of fingering worry beads.

You will have seen these curious beads nestled in the hands of Arab sheikhs. If you'd followed the stockmarket boom in the 1980s, you may have seen a prominent stockbroker carrying a solid gold string of them.

These Middle Eastern worry beads have their Indian and Western counterparts, too. Have you ever wondered what Hare Krishnas carry in that little bag that covers their left hand? And more than one Western religion uses rosary beads for keeping place during contemplative prayer rituals, while monks and certain religious orders even use them as part of their tunics.

What does all this have to do with you finding relief from stress?

Worry beads work. They are a fast, simple, little technique for dealing with stress.

The act of fingering them uses up the nervous energy in your fingers. The slow, repetitive passage of beads through your fidgety little fingers, with little or no physical and intellectual effort required, is surprisingly soothing. Moreover, if you use these beads for extended periods – say 30 minutes to an hour at a time – the effect can be almost meditative. In fact, if you perform this little exercise with complete concentration, it becomes a meditation.

To use them, first find yourself a string of 20–30 chickpea-sized beads. Their origin is unimportant, as is their design.

If you want to follow tradition, hold them in your left hand. Using your thumb and forefinger, slowly finger your way through the beads.

Concentrate on doing this as smoothly and as effortlessly as possible. If you do this for some time, you will become aware of nothing but them and the fact that you are using them. This is, in effect, a calming meditative state and is one of the calmest states you will achieve.

The Way of the Tree

If I were to tell you that spending 30 minutes alone wandering through a leafy park or garden would do more towards reducing your stress levels than any drug or stimulant, you'd say, 'Big deal, everyone knows that'.

It's true, everyone does know it. But how many people do you know who will turn to this shortcut to peace and tranquillity at times of tension and anxiety?

Walking in a visually pleasing, oxygen-rich environment like a park has an immediate and measurable effect on our stress levels. Do it twice a day and you would be well on the way to being a very calm person.

Moreover, if the views you're taking in are of a long-distance variety (distant mountains, sprawling valleys, rolling seas), then the benefit is even more pronounced. Because views such as this fill us with feelings of openness and hope.

But what if no such views are available or no park is nearby? What if you cannot leave your workplace during the day?

If this is the case, you have two powerful alternatives.

The first is simply to imagine yourself in such an environment. Use the techniques from the Big Screen Visualisation on page 94. Just by concentrating on the required image, and by placing yourself in it, you will discover a real sense of calm.

The second technique is one that's been popular in Japan for centuries. It's the miniature garden. A meditation garden, if you like.

In Japan, where outdoor space is at a premium, these gardens are both tiny and understated, usually taking up no more space than your average cabbage patch. Yet, because they depend more on imagination than they do on your physical presence, their power to soothe is immense.

Building on the belief that even the smallest glimpse of nature is sometimes all that you need to release you from the pressures and anxieties of everyday life, you can bring this 'meditation garden' experience right into your home or office. With a miniature Japanese garden. You'll get most of the concepts and all of the materials from any good bonsai shop.

Even the creation of your own little patch of nature will be soothing.

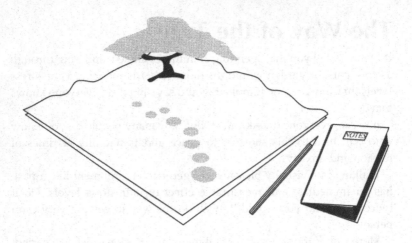

Then, when it's completed, all you have to do is sit somewhere quiet and concentrate on it for 10–15 minutes. It depends on your commitment to the illusion, but many of those who've tried this miniature meditation garden have been astounded at the peace and comfort it can bring.

(You can make this experience even more effective by enhancing it with New Age recordings of nature – birds, running streams and so on – available from many record stores. Combine this with meditative thoughts and you will have a most powerful combination at your disposal.)

Stress Ball

Before the days of Nautilus body-building machines, a popular wrist-strengthening device consisted a plain ball that was squeezed in the hand. The idea was that this was a non-gym exercise to be repeatedly performed at any place, at any time of the day or night.

You might recall seeing these 'squeeze balls' being used in movies from the late Fifties – for a while, it became a bit of a Hollywood cliché for uptight, macho characters to go about squeezing them all the time. While there were balls specifically designed for this exercise, the common squash ball was an all-purpose substitute.

Many people who participated in this curious exercise discovered an interesting and unexpected byproduct. As well as developing wrist strength, the squeeze ball was also a great relaxant and reliever of tension. This mindless, repetitive exercise was almost meditative in its effect, working in a manner not unlike worry beads, basket weaving or knitting would work for others.

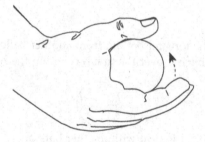

Figure 67

This same exercise can work for you. In fact, there is a burgeoning market today for 'stress balls' – similar sized balls filled with various squishy substances – that you squeeze throughout the day to relieve the tensions that build in your body and concentrate in your hands.

But it's just as easy to make one yourself.

DO-IT-YOURSELF STRESS BALL

Cut the stem from a small water balloon.

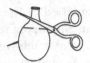

Fill with rice or lentils.

Cut the top and bottom from another balloon and
stretch it over the first – covering the hole.

Repeat with another balloon.

Repeat with as many more as it takes to be
aesthetically pleasing to you.

Now squeeze away to your heart's content.

Chinese Palm Balls

It is said that these date from the Ming Dynasty (AD 1368–1644) where they were originally designed to build strength – not unlike the Western 'squeeze balls' favoured by Charles Bronson.

These Chinese Palm Balls – known by a variety of names, some as exotic as 'Double Balls of Roaring Dragon and Singing Phoenix' – are made from steel or brass and are about the size of a golf ball, or larger. They have evolved over the centuries into the hollowed-out version with soundboard inside that you will find in Chinatown today, resting in silk-lined cases.

When handled gently, these palm balls emit a tone, almost like a chime, that has been attributed with all kinds of miraculous claims ranging from the prevention of arthritis to the cure of hypertension.

I prefer not to attempt to validate these claims, other than to say that they do work on the acupressure points of the hand. I can also attest to the reputation of Chinese Palm Balls as a device that is most effective in soothing the nerves. If you use them as described, they can have a uniquely calming influence.

CHINESE PALM BALLS

- Remember the Conditions of Calm.
- Commence Power Breathing.
- Hold two or more Chinese Palm Balls in the palm of your right hand. Using all of your fingers, move the balls in a counter-clockwise direction.
- Repeat in a clockwise direction in your left hand.

Flax Pack

What if there were a device that harnessed the advantages of some of the acupressure techniques we have covered earlier, yet required no physical effort on your part as it soothed away the stresses and strains of everyday life?

Such a device is the Flax Pack.

In essence, it is nothing more than a silk blackout that presses gently on the eyes; in practice, it is a massage device that caresses many of the acupressure points that reside in this area.

The construction of the Flax Pack is simplicity itself: a satin silk bag filled with flax seeds (linseeds). Cool silk combined with firm, but pliable, flax seeds add up to a remarkably soothing eye press – a unique package of smoothness, firmness, coolness and sensuousness.

To use it, you simply lie back in a comfortable place, drape the Flax Pack across your closed eyes, and let its cool, gentle pressure soothe away your stresses – almost instantly. While in this restful position, you can apply any of the other techniques from this book, particularly Power Breathing.

TO CONSTRUCT A FLAX PACK

- Take a piece of satin silk, 18 cm (7 in) square. Fold it in half, and stitch together two of the sides, leaving the top open.
- Turn inside out.
- Fill with 200 g (7 oz) of natural linseeds, taking care not to overfill. Sew up the top of the pack.
- In warm weather, leave the Flax Pack in the refrigerator for 20 minutes before using to make it even more soothing.
- Add a few drops of lavender or rose essential oil.

Float Tank

Strange but wonderful stress relief devices reached their zenith in the Seventies with the introduction of the float tank. Initially dismissed as a bit weird and Californian, the float tank enjoyed only limited popularity until interest was reawakened in the high-stress Eighties.

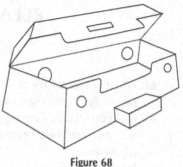

Figure 68

Although they come in all shapes and specifications, the float tank is – at its most basic – a light-proof fibreglass tank half filled with a saline solution.

In theory, it is the world's easiest stress-release exercise: you climb in, lower the lid and, floating on your back, dissolve away your stress. The highly salinated (salted) water means you float easily, and the light-proof, sound-proof environment removes all distraction.

In practice, the float tank has a few drawbacks. For a start, it is expensive: to be effective, it needs to be used regularly, yet it can cost as much as a full massage. Even though the average tank is quite large, many users find them claustrophobic. And, if you're not used to wearing ear plugs, you may find the sensation of floating on your back, with your ears beneath water level, a little disconcerting.

For those who persist, however, the float tank can be a unique tool for deep relaxation.

Floating is a pleasant and effortless way of removing almost all the physical stress from your body. The complete absence of stimuli – absolute darkness, your ears beneath water level blocking out all external sound – allows you to eliminate distractions in a way that many meditators would envy. Indeed, this absence of external stimuli forces your concentration inward so that you can easily focus on the sound of your own breathing.

Some aficionados have relaxation or self-improvement sound tracks piped into the float tank itself, believing that in those conditions the subconscious is in a more receptive state (which it is). You can also perform a progressive relaxation technique (see box overleaf).

FLOAT TANK PROGRESSIVE RELAXATION

- When you enter the tank spend a few minutes performing Power Breathing exercises.
- Feel your hands floating gently float on the water. Ensure that they are completely relaxed and hold no tension whatsoever.
- Imagine that floating feeling seeping from your hands to your elbows, along your arms, into your shoulders.
- Imagine that floating feeling spreading from your shoulders, across your back, up the back of your neck.
- Imagine that floating feeling spreading down your back, into your buttocks and thighs, down to your feet.
- Now reverse this procedure, letting that floating feeling work up from your feet all the way to your hands.
- Concentrate on the sound of your breathing (which will be more pronounced than usual since you are wearing ear plugs).

Whichever way it is used, the float tank experience falls into one of two categories: it will quickly relieve your stressful feelings, or it will have the opposite effect. Only experience will tell.

But if you try it and it works for you, floating can be an effortless and fascinating way to relieve the stresses of modern life.

D.I.Y. Float Tank

A low-cost alternative to the float tank is one well within your reach. It takes place in your own bathroom – assuming that your bathroom is a reasonably quiet and warm room with a sizeable tub.

At the core of this technique is a warm bath. Warm water – a few degrees warmer than your normal body temperature – has a powerful relaxing effect: it increases blood circulation, relaxes the muscles and, according to recent theory, induces biochemical changes that actually tranquillise. (Avoid water that is too hot as it shocks the system and causes the muscles to contract.)

To create the float tank effect, simply pour a packet of Epsom Salts into the warm water (creating the saline solution). For added benefits, you might also consider adding a few drops of calming essential oils. Once you have done this, light a candle or turn out the lights. Then, when you are comfortably immersed in the water, commence Power Breathing and perform the Float Tank Progressive Relaxation exercises.

Fork and Spade

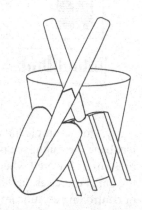

Take a walk through the suburbs and take note of the calm and unstressed people you see. What do they have in common? Are they joggers? Picnickers? Shoppers?

So often they'll be gardeners. A whole lot more good comes out of the garden than nutrition. Gardeners are often among the most calm and relaxed people (while they're gardening) you'll find, because gardening is one of the most natural stress-releasing activities you'll find.

One can speculate on the reasons for this, but the obvious is that you're working with the earth, you're doing something physical and, most important of all, you're doing something constructive – not something contrived like working out at a health club.

Then, as a reward for your labours, you create your own haven of peace and tranquillity with vegetables, flowers, trees or even pebbles.

Bio-feedback

About the same time of the rise of the float tank, and of Timothy Leary and LSD in the USA, a high-tech means of achieving deep meditative states came back into prominence.

In its most well-known application it was known as bio-feedback.

Bio-feedback is usually an electronic way of regulating physiological processes that, ordinarily, cannot be voluntarily regulated. Using a variety of measuring devices – such as electrodes taped to the chest, skull or elsewhere – you can teach yourself to regulate functions like blood pressure, heart beat, muscle spasm, pain, even brain waves.

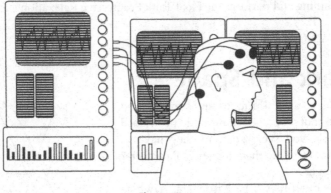

Figure 69

Say, for example, a man has high blood pressure. Using bio-feedback, he might see on the monitor in front of him how his blood pressure is lowered when he thinks of floating clouds – or of performing ballet exercises. In this way, bio-feedback can teach him a technique of controlling an 'uncontrollable', such as his own blood pressure.

Bio-feedback can also function in this way to control stress and anxiety. However, to understand how it works as a stress-control device, you need to know a little about how meditation works.

Meditation produces a state of deep relaxation where, unlike sleep, your mind is wide awake and alert. During the meditative state, there is a unique change in the pattern of your brain waves. There is an increase in alpha waves – usually only present when you are wide awake and relaxed. And there is an increase in delta waves – usually only present in the deepest sleep.

The paradox of meditation is that alpha and delta waves – indicating wide awake and deep sleep – are present at the same time. By all conventional physiological standards, this should be impossible.

Conventionally, bio-feedback's role as a calm device means concentrating on alpha waves only. Using a variety of technical methods, you use your own conscious mind to regulate the alpha waves your brain produces. When you produce sufficient alpha waves, a state of relaxation follows. That's all there is to it.

While bio-feedback sometimes takes several sessions to master, a user eventually becomes adept at producing deep states of relaxation simply by being tuned in to the pattern of his or her own brain waves!

Meditation Goggles

In recent years, the bio-feedback concept has spawned a number of electronic devices specially designed for combating stress.

Most of the types I am familiar with use variations on sound and light to stimulate certain physiological responses. One of the more intriguing of these devices is variously known as meditation goggles or as a wave synchroniser.

Broadly, this consists of a small programming unit, from which a pair of goggles, and sometimes headphones, are wired. The principle is that by varying light pulses in the goggles and sound pulses in the headphones you can influence the alpha waves produced by the brain. And, by increasing the alpha waves, you enter a state of deep relaxation and creativity.

While the principle behind Meditation Goggles appears reasonably sound, how does it work in practice? I know of many who swear by it. Equally as many, however, find the electronic nature of such a device to be both intrusive and aesthetically unsound.

Try it. It could be the easiest way yet of discovering real calm.

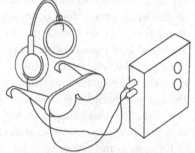

Figure 70

Calm Music

Music soothes the savage breast, as William Congreve claimed, but does it really reduce stress levels? Can music, by itself, help you move from an anxious state to a more peaceful one? I'm sure most of us believe that it can do this.

Music therapists now know that music can effect real physiological change, not only in the obvious areas of heart beat and breathing rhythm, but in galvanic skin response, blood pressure, hormone levels, immune response and brain wave activity – all of which relate to our feelings of stress and anxiety.

Recent studies have shown that calming music played in operating theatres can induce a more relaxed state in the patient and thus reduce the amount of anaesthetic required during an operation. Similarly, if you've ever listened to Debussy through headphones while you're in the dentist's chair, you will appreciate how beneficial that can be in the reduction of pain or the fear of pain. Music therapists (yes, they exist) now know that music can have a profound effect in limiting our feelings of stress and anxiety.

But what sort of music does it take? And how should you use it?

Obviously, the music should be slow, quiet and instrumental; lyrics, unless especially written to soothe, are best avoided since they can have a stimulating effect instead. But over and above all else, the most elementary requirements for soothing music are familiarity and personal taste: it's no use playing Bach if your taste dictates Basie.

My research has shown, however, that the ideal calm music has a tempo slightly slower than your heart beat – this encourages your pulse rate to slow down to match; sometimes this even lowers blood pressure at the same time. Most commercial music tends to be considerably faster than this, so it may pay to visit the Classics, the Romantics, or any slow jazz pieces (being wary of the blues). I read in *Rolling Stone* once that the two music forms that created 'positive vibrations' were classical and reggae. Unfortunately, I have not been able to corroborate the latter – though the slow rhythm of some reggae pieces may fulfil this objective – and suspect it has as much to do with marijuana haze and Bob Marley's claims as it does with reality.

Rhythm is not the only criterion of calm music, of course. Melody can be equally as important.

Experiment.

Listen to Erik Satie's *Gymnopédies*, or Chopin's *Nocturnes*, Shostakovich's *Symphony No. 10*, Saint-Saëns's *Allegro Appassionato* or *Le Cygne*, Delius's *Romance*, Elgar's *Salut d'Amour*, Fauré's *Après un Rêve*, Schubert's *Symphony No. 8 in B Minor 'Unfinished'*, Debussy's *Trois Nocturnes*, Bach's *Concerto in D minor for Two Violins*. Alternatively, listen to some of Dexter Gordon's early tenor saxophone, or even some of Charlie Mingus's slower works.

If you can't find anything that works for you, try one of the many 'meditation music' or 'New Age' tapes on the market: you're sure to find something in that category that works for you (even though I find most of it rather clichéd and uninspiring, it generally works as a 'mood setter' for most of the other techniques in this book).

Finally, if music fails to satisfy, consider a light breeze and a set of wind chimes. For some, there is nothing more soothing than the random melodies that only the breeze can inspire. (Naturally, the unpredictable nature of the breeze is the limiting factor in this technique.) If you do decide to follow this course, the type of chimes is important – for my taste, the most soothing materials are bamboo or, oddly enough, aluminium.

CALM MUSIC

- Find a quiet place and sit comfortably with your eyes closed, listening to your chosen music.
- Commence Power Breathing.
- After a minute or so, turn your attention from your breathing to the music.
- Give yourself over to the music. Try to 'feel' the notes as they come in contact with your body; try to 'see' them as they wash over you.
- The more you can 'feel' or 'see' the notes, the more the stress and tension in your body will dissolve.

Hypno-melodic Themes

For years now, since I wrote *the Calm Technique,* I have searched for a music accompaniment that would encourage the deeper levels of relaxation.

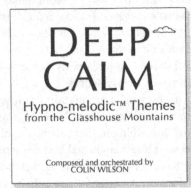

Even though I did come across a number of tapes and albums that purported to be this, I found them to be a little contrived and self-conscious. Those which were real and impressive tended to be a little distracting because of their musicality.

Then two years ago I discovered a group of musicians in Queensland's Glasshouse Mountains (a mystical place if ever there was one) performing an unusual kind of music they called Mud Music.

Although it was originally commissioned to accompany a pottery exhibition, it had a hypnotic quality quite unlike anything I'd ever experienced before. Indeed, there have since been articles on this Mud Music in the international music press.

As a result of this experience, I suggested a composition designed expressly to produce a state of deep relaxation in untrained listeners. The result of this is a new type of music called *Hypno-Melodic Themes.* It has been especially conceived, composed and arranged to produce profound states of relaxation.

I commend this music to you as one of the few meditation tracks that, for me, really works. It is deceptively simple, but very powerful. Any serious student of relaxation or meditation should at least give it an audition.

(You should be able to find *Hypno-Melodic Themes* at your record store. If not, you may order a compact disc by writing to The Calm Centre, PO Box 404, Northbridge, New South Wales 2063, Australia.)

Listen in peace.

Guatemalan Worry Doll

For many, one of the most effective techniques for dispensing with worry is one that was developed hundreds, perhaps thousands, of years ago in the rainforests of Guatemala.

The children of these areas used an ingenious little device for handling the traumas of the day and for containing their childish concerns and worries. So effective was it in achieving this that, as these children grew older, many of them used the same device to contain adult worries.

The device is known as the Guatemalan Worry Doll. This is not a doll as you know it, nor does it look like a little Guatemalan baby. Indeed, these dolls often have no human resemblance at all. What they look like, however, is unimportant; what they enable you to do is all that matters.

Essentially, the Guatemalan Worry Doll is a miniature basket with a removable lid. Inside are one or several 'dolls', which may be rough pieces of twig, or complex little carved characters, or anything in between – the design has no bearing on the effectiveness of the package.

The way it works is childlike in its simplicity, yet elegant in its psychology.

If, during the day, a Guatema-lan child is beset by a worry or worries, she simply lifts the lid before going to bed and whispers her concern to the 'doll' inside. The doll is then left to do the worrying overnight while the child sleeps peacefully and untroubled.

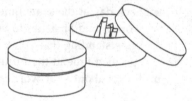

Figure 71

Ingenious? Weird? Naive? Perhaps all three. But it does work. The issue is, how can we make it work for you?

You can make a Guatemalan Worry Doll yourself out of any object – a cotton reel, a purple crystal, a plain old envelope. In itself, it has no particularly important form, design or properties.

What is more important is your faith in your ability to transfer your anxieties elsewhere. 'Transferring your anxieties' is obviously a meta-phor for simply dismissing them from your mind. And, taking into account that it is the subconscious mind that will perform this task – the part of your mind that enthusiastically responds to images and metaphors – you can see how feasible this might be ... regardless of the childlike nature of the device that facilitates it.

Moreover, if you employ this technique in a regular, ritualised way, you can make certain that it will work for you. You will be able to transfer your anxieties (that is, dismiss them from your mind) in a regular, ritualised way.

Those Guatemalan children really knew what they were doing.

THE GUATEMALAN WORRY DOLL

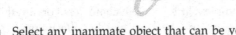

- Select any inanimate object that can be your Guatemalan Worry Doll.
- It does not need to be anything even resembling a doll. A cotton reel or envelope would suffice.
- Each day at the same time, in the same place, whisper your worries and anxieties to your 'worry doll'. Do this in the understanding that you will take them up again at some specified time in the future (e.g. tomorrow).
- Forget about your worries and anxieties for the time being.

The Ioniser

There are sceptics about who scoff at the effectiveness of ionisers in the house. They are wrong! They are unbelievably wrong.

These days, the ioniser is a common contraption in aware households. Its real name is a negative ion generator – because its total function in life is to generate negative ions.

Contrary to the superficial reading of the word, negative ions have a very positive effect. They freshen the air, they assist your breathing and, most especially, they induce a feeling calm and energy at the same time.

Even if you don't have an ioniser of your own, you will have already experienced the effects of negative ions. In those moments preceding and following electrical storms, the air is charged with these blessed little particles. When they're present, you will find it easier to breathe and the air will seem cleaner, almost cool to the 'touch'. Many people find these conditions to be refreshing, mood-enhancing, even uplifting.

And, guess what! The air *is* much cleaner. Dust particles become electrically charged in the storms and are taken out of the atmosphere. This is why dust and soot gathers around your ioniser if you leave it turned on for extended periods. This is why recording studies and computer rooms often install commercial ionisers to protect their sensitive equipment.

The ioniser is a low-cost device that reproduces this electrical storm atmospheric condition. Place one beside your bed, or beside your computer, and you will breeze through the day or night feeling better and more relaxed.

How?

It accomplishes this because negative ions stimulate the production of *serotonin* in the brain. (Serotonin is the transmitter that causes slow-wave sleep.) In other words, there are sound physiological reasons why negative ions really do make you feel more relaxed.

Use one and you'll never look back.

The Pet

For centuries now, stressed people have known the virtues of a remarkably appealing, and highly effective, antidote to the stresses of everyday life.

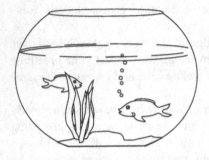

A pet.

Numerous studies have shown that people who share their lives with a pet not only suffer less from the effects of stress and anxiety, but are also better able to deal with each occurrence of it. Indeed, some studies indicate that keeping a pet can actually increase your lifespan.

It is not difficult to understand why. With a pet we can be completely natural; we play with them, cuddle them, talk to them, even confide in them – and they never judge or criticise. And as long as we treat them reasonably well, they believe each of us is the most wonderful being ever created.

And that can be a bonus when you're striving to feel calm.

Calm Wardrobe

Back in the Sixties, did the hippies know something ordinary people did not? Does the Arab bedouin, the Indian yogi and the Buddhist monk understand a principle of calm that followers of fashion do not?

Indeed they do. They know how important garments can be to their state of mind.

Several years back, when researching *the Calm Technique* in a number of rather esoteric meditation centres, I learned that clothing could play a major influence on the way you felt. Light-coloured clothes made you feel more peaceful than dark. Loose clothes made you feel more relaxed than tight. Cotton made you feel more peaceful than synthetics.

A loose, white, cotton garment, therefore, would have a powerful effect on how calm you could be feeling. Or, according to the cognoscenti, loose cotton garments dyed with vegetable or mineral dyes will have you feeling calmer than synthetic dyes.

In discussing this with my colleagues, I found opinions leaned to two extremes – one group insisted this was purely psychosomatic, while the other was prepared to accept that there *could* be some physical attribute to these colours, styles and fabrics that really did influence the way you felt. I suspect they were both right.

I also know that it doesn't really matter one way or the other, because such clothes do influence the way you feel! So if you want to feel calm and more relaxed, simply choose loose-fitting, light-coloured, natural fibres. I do.

Massage Sandal

Because we spend most of our days walking on hard and unforgiving surfaces, in hard and unforgiving shoes, it is little wonder that our feet are the source of so many physical difficulties. Not only can these contribute to problems and discomfort in the legs, but they can cause problems in the lower back area as well.

This encourages stressful feelings throughout the body.

A simple way around this condition is the massage sandal. With these sandals, you walk about on scores of little rubber 'spikes' and immediately begin to ease the aches and pains from your feet and legs.

More importantly, though, these spikes correspond with the acupressure points at the base of the foot and, through constant massage of these points as you walk or stand, a feeling of relaxation is encouraged throughout the entire body. It takes a couple of weeks of discomfort for your feet to adjust, but this is well worth the perseverance.

The Splint

It is a sobering statistic that something as common as a clamped jaw (tensed jaw muscles) can be the source of so many of stress-related complaints, particularly those that centre around the head area. The ailments it causes range from headaches to painfully stiff necks, to generalised feelings of unease. (The reasons for this are explained more fully on page 29 where I examined the phenomenon of referred pain.)

Oddly enough, the therapist who can work wonders in relieving the pressures that build in this area has nothing to do with alternative healing – it's your dentist.

If you suffer from a clenched jaw and tight masseter (jaw) muscles in this way, ask your dentist about a little dental prosthetic called a 'splint' or a 'de-programmer'. This simple device is worn over the back teeth and is particularly effective at reducing the urge to clench your teeth which, in turn, reduces much of the muscular tension in the jaw area.

This, in turn, prevents the spread of muscular tension throughout your skull, neck and shoulders.

(A lower cost, and more readily available, alternative to the splint is the Jaw Release technique on page 126–7.)

Barber's Towel

When it comes to relaxation, what do barber shops, beauty therapists, the first-class sections of many airlines and Japanese restaurants have in common?

They all know the soothing powers of the hot towel.

It does not require a wealth of skill to perfect the art of preparing a hot towel. And to apply this soothing age-old technique, simply take a small face towel or washer, immerse it in warm to hot water, then wring it out. Then all you have to do is drape it over your face, and sit back with your eyes closed.

You'll be surprised at how fast the tension drains from your body and how soon you'll be relaxed. Combine a hot towel with any of the other techniques in this book, and your path to feeling calm and relaxed is made even more pleasurable.

THE BARBER'S TOWEL

- Soak a small towel in warm to hot water, then wring it out.
- Recline in a quiet place. Remember the Conditions of Calm.
- Close your eyes and place the hot towel over your face.
- Perform Power Breathing exercises as you lie back and relax.

22

CALM FOODS, HERBS AND POTIONS

Calm Vitamins

Vitamins play a major role in the way you handle stress as well as your susceptibility to it. But how do you determine which vitamins you need as well as the quantities you need them in?

The manufacturers of vitamin supplements usually advise that vitamins may be useful only if you have an inadequate intake through your regular diet. That level is generally accepted to be a figure published by regulatory bodies of various types around the world, known as the Recommended Daily Dietary Allowances. These figures are frequently disputed by vitamin therapists who insist that different people and different conditions require different levels, and that even environmental factors greatly affect these requirements.

Take vitamin E, or example. People on diets high in unsaturated fats have a greater need than 'normal' for vitamin E. Similarly, those who have a high dependence on bread and cereals in their diets will be missing out on a major source of vitamin E if these foodstuffs are made from processed, rather than wholegrain, products.

More pertinent to the interests of this book, your ability to produce pituitary and adrenal hormones (which assist in the handling of stress, and are severely depleted by it) is dependent on a correct balance of vitamins in your diet. A deficiency in vitamin E, the B vitamins or vitamin A limits your body's manufacture of these 'anti-stress' hormones.

CALM VITAMINS

As a general principle, for 'calm vitamin' consumption, choose as many foods as possible from the following.

- **Vitamin E foods**: most vegetables (especially raw), many fruits, eggs, dairy products.

- **Vitamin A foods** (which counter the negative effects of stress): yoghurt, cream, butter, eggs, liver, carrots, leafy green vegetables, fruit.

- **Vitamin C foods** (which have a positive effect on your mental health): all fruit and vegetables, some of the best sources being capsicum, blackcurrants, kiwifruit, Brussels sprouts, strawberries, orange.

- **Magnesium foods**: wholegrain flour and cereals, seeds.

- **Pantothenic acid (vitamin B5) foods**: peanuts, cabbage, cauliflower, broccoli, liver, eggs.

- **Other vitamin B foods**: beans, lentils, peas, nuts, seeds, wheatgerm, bran, wholegrains, milk, cheese, yoghurt, meat, fish, poultry and green leafy vegetables. (Remember the B vitamins, like most vitamins, are rapidly diminished by light, heat, steam, long cooking and long storage.)

As well, any deficiency in your vitamin C intake means a corresponding increase in your susceptibility to physical or emotional stress. (Also, there have been recent studies that say magnesium – a mineral, not a vitamin – is a useful antidote to the ill-effects of stress.)

Vitamins C, E, A and some of the B vitamins are known as 'antioxidants', and are believed by many to have powerful healing, calming and anti-aging qualities.

Knowing what vitamins you need is one thing; maintaining their correct levels is quite something else.

The ideal is to get them through your normal dietary intake. This is not always practical, perhaps not even achievable. However if your dietary intake is inadequate, vitamin supplements are readily available.

It should be noted that pregnant women are always advised to seek further medical advice before adopting any extreme vitamin therapies.

Calm Foods

Nowadays, it's common enough knowledge that diet affects your emotions and mental state as much as it does your body. To resort to a cliché, you really are what you eat.

But is it possible that certain foods can be described as 'calm foods', and that these foods can have a soothing effect on your stress or anxiety levels? You'd better believe it.

Whether certain foods will have an instant effect on these states, however, is a matter for experiment. Some will be immediate, others will take 30 minutes or so, others may take considerably longer. But they will have an effect!

If you doubt this, I urge you to try the following: spend one whole day eating nothing but raw vegetables and fruit. Ensure these are the only foodstuffs you consume during this day – in whatever quantities, in whatever combination you choose.

At the end of 12 or so hours you will feel more calm and relaxed. Nothing is surer.

If you're normally a heavy eater, particularly a heavy meat eater, you may not feel terribly sated – at least not the first time you try this – but you *will* feel more calm and in control!

(This is not necessarily my recommendation for your ongoing diet, but it will demonstrate the calming properties of certain foods.)

Acids and alkalines for calm

There are two types of foods in any diet: acid-forming foods and alkaline-forming foods. The ideal calm diet maintains a ratio of alkalines to acids of about 80:20.

Upsetting this ratio in favour of the acids – that is, consuming too many acid-producing foods – contributes not only to illness, but to feelings of stress.

Conversely, consuming greater proportions of alkaline foods, particularly at stressful times, will help you cope better.

Alkaline-forming foods (ideally 80 per cent of your diet) are: wholegrain flour and cereals, fruits, vegetables, especially uncooked.

Acid-forming foods (ideally 20 per cent of your diet) are: coffee, meat, sugar, processed foods, white flour, nuts, preservatives.

Maintain this ratio of 80:20 and you will be well on the way to nullifying the negative effects of stress.

Here is a list of foods that have special properties for anyone contemplating a Calm Diet.

Sprouts   Sprouts are one of nature's wonder foods. They are superb sources of the B vitamins and vitamin C – all useful vitamins in the treatment of stress-related conditions. (The vitamin B2 content of oats, for example, increases up to 2000 per cent after they've been sprouted.)

Bananas   To handle stress well, you need to maintain a correct balance between sodium and potassium in your diet. In most diets, the balance invariably weighs in favour of sodium (salt). By limiting your salt intake, and by eating more potassium foods, such as bananas, you can correct that balance. Potassium also encourages respiration and oxygenation in the bloodstream, both of which contribute to you feeling more relaxed and in control.

In two dietary experiments I know of, bananas have been associated with feelings of increased energy, as well as a sense of cheerfulness and wellbeing. Too many can be fattening though (they're the favoured diet of sumo wrestlers).

Liver   Whilst it should be consumed in moderation, and does not suit every tastebud or diet, liver is one of the richest sources of vitamins A and B-complex, and contains significant levels of magnesium, all of which are essential to reversing the effects of stress.

Kiwifruit Known for their high vitamin C content (many times more than in an orange), the kiwifruit is also a rich source of potassium.

Tomatoes Yet another rich source of potassium (about 400 mg in an average one) is the tomato, especially if it is vine-ripened. If you add fresh **basil** or **tarragon**, both of which are known for their relaxing properties, you have a doubly effective dish, *particularly if the tomatoes are uncooked.*

Beans (dried) Another great source of potassium and, as a result, they have good calming properties. Lima and soybeans are the best. **Tofu**, which is made from soybeans, is also worthy of inclusion in your diet.

Eggs The cholesterol scare has done a lot of harm to the reputation of the humble egg. Today's thinking, however, is not as condemning as it used to be. In fact, many dietitians now encourage their use – not surprising when eggs are such a great source of vitamins E, B2, A and D.

Wheatgerm There is no richer source of vitamin E than wheatgerm. It is also rich in magnesium.

Sesame seeds An excellent source of vitamins E and B-complex and magnesium.

Yoghurt Rich in B-complex vitamins as well as vitamins A and D, all of which are invaluable in countering the effects of stress. Reduced-fat yoghurt contains less vitamins than whole-milk yoghurt.

Oats A rich source of vitamin B2, and many say they have calming properties far in excess of their vitamin levels. I believe they are one of the most important foods for anyone who lives a stressful life.

The Calm Diet

It may come as no surprise to you to learn that the ideal diet is a balanced one rich in vegetables, fruits, complex carbohydrates and wholegrains, but low in fats. Not only does such a diet maintain your calm, but provides maximum energy and a sense of wellbeing throughout the day.

Wherever possible, start your day with fresh fruit or fruit juice, and begin each meal with raw vegetables or a salad.

Use fruit or wholegrain bread as snack foods, and you will feel better for it in all possible ways.

Wherever possible, avoid the 'quick fixes': coffee, soft drinks, sugar and fat-laden snack foods. While these may elevate your mood momentarily, they will encourage both tension and lethargy within a very short time.

THE CALM DIET

As a general principle, **choose** the following foodstuffs:

- more fruit and vegetables, especially raw ones
- yoghurt, milk, cream, butter, eggs
- wholegrain cereals and breads
- beans, lentils, peas, nuts, seeds, wheatgerm, bran
- meat, fish, poultry (in moderation).

As a general principle, **avoid** the following foodstuffs:

- artificial additives of all kinds
- excessive sugar, salt and spices
- refined foods
- preserved foods.

Adherents of some of the traditional meditation disciplines insist that foods can be divided into distinct categories, each of which has an effect on the emotional state. Experimentation with these foods does tend to confirm many of their beliefs.

According to yogic principles, all foods fall into three categories: 'calm foods', 'stimulating foods' and 'lethargic foods'. To be calm and relaxed, the ideal dietary combination would consist mostly of calm foods, with minimal stimulating foods and no lethargic foods.

Calm foods

These are easily digested, cleansing, calming and provide maximum energy. They include:

- all kinds of fruits
- most vegetables (with as little cooking as possible)
- nuts and seeds in their natural state
- beans
- grains
- milk and milk products (shunned by the Chinese, revered by the Indians)
- herbs and spices (in moderation).

Stimulating foods

These foods create unrest and heightened activity in the mind. In the yogic diet, they are consumed only in the most modest proportions. They include:

- excessive spices
- vinegar
- radishes, garlic and onion
- coffee, tea, cola
- all foods with preservatives
- most canned and packaged foods.

Lethargic foods

In the yogic diet, these are the foods to be avoided. They demand too much time and energy to digest, and create feelings of inertia. Some of them also fall into the previous category of stimulating foods. Meat, as an example, causes feelings of lethargy and tiredness as well as a general feeling of restlessness. Lethargic foods include:

- meats of all kinds
- refined foods
- alcohol
- fermented (e.g. pickled) or stale foods.

You will probably recognise the above as a basic vegetarian wholefood diet – not at all uncommon in this day and age. Whether you choose to follow it, or simply to integrate some of its underlying principles into your usual diet, is not for this book to suggest.

What *is* important, though, is that you appreciate how real a role different foods play in the way you feel. By choosing them carefully, you can certainly help yourself feel calm and relaxed.

Migraine foods

While we're on the topic of foods, it might be worth considering the foodstuffs that are known to aggravate migraine conditions in many sufferers. Generally, these foods contain either tyramine, nitrate, monosodium glutamate or alcohol. The most common of these are:

- chocolate
- cheese, yoghurt, sour cream
- eggs
- pork, bacon, ham, sausage
- pickled foods
- wheat and gluten products
- peanuts
- tomatoes, broad beans
- citrus fruits
- alcohol.

Calm Drinks

Interestingly, there is perhaps a greater number of fluids that will have an immediate calming effect on you than there are foods.

At the very top of that list, the most calming drink of them all is chamomile tea.

Chamomile   Once considered the drink of 'alternative folk', chamomile tea is now widely accepted as the drink that brings on sleepiness.

But chamomile tea has an even more useful function as an instant antidote to stress. Keep a packet of it around at all times, and when stressful situations arise have a chamomile instead of an ordinary (caffeine including) tea. The effect will be so pronounced you might wonder why there's any need for the rest of this book.

If the taste doesn't appeal, add a little honey or lemon, or a pinch of peppermint tea at the same time.

Other herbal teas known for their calming effects are lime blossom, orange blossom, passion flower, wood betony, lavender, possibly rose hip and hibiscus.

Celery juice   Also has powerful calming properties. Celery is a member of the parsley family and contains a unique sedative compound, panthalide. One glass of celery juice (combine it with carrot juice if you prefer) is not only refreshing, but will make you feel considerably more relaxed within minutes.

Blackcurrant juice   A rich source of gamma-linolenic acid (GLA) which is said to be effective for the treatment of hypertension and lowering of blood pressure. It encourages feelings of calm. Blackcurrant also contains high levels of vitamin C.

Peppermint   Although known more as a digestive aid, peppermint has significant calming properties. If you substitute peppermint herbal tea for more stimulating drinks such as coffee and tea, the effects on your emotional state are multiplied many times.

Dandelion   There are a number of coffee substitutes made from dandelion root (which contains mannitol, a useful substance for treating hypertension and feelings of anxiety). You will find them in health food stores. If you substitute this dandelion drink for coffee, the calming effects are multiplied once again.

Milk Milk contains an amino acid called tryptophan that the body converts to serotonin; this triggers the deepest level of sleep in the brain. Furthermore, milk is high in calcium, which is widely regarded as a muscle relaxant. So the old adage of 'a glass of milk before bedtime makes you sleep more soundly' has a real scientific basis.

Chai One of the most popular drinks in India, chai, is also one of the more calming. Two of its ingredients – milk and ginger – have known calming properties. To make this refreshing drink bring one cup of milk and one cup of water to the boil together, add tea, a cinnamon stick, sugar (or honey) and a few good-sized slices of ginger, and allow to draw for 5 minutes. Some add a pinch of black pepper as well, but you may find this and the sugar a little too stimulating.

TO MAKE HERBAL TEA

By far the most convenient way to make a herbal tea is to drop in a tea bag. Some teas, however, are not available in bags. And just as some people prefer 'real' tea to tea bags, others prefer 'real' herbal infusions.

The simplest way to make a herbal tea from real herbs is to place a teaspoon of the fresh or dried herbs in a pot, cover with hot water, then let sit for 5–10 minutes.

To increase the taste appeal of some teas, you can add a slice of lemon or a little honey. Also, teas like peppermint and rosehip make refreshing drinks when chilled.

Magic Water

Water is the basis of all life. The human body is made up primarily of water. The food we eat is made up primarily of water (yes, even a cooked steak is 70 per cent water). And, along with air, the element we cannot survive without for long is water.

An adequate intake of water enhances many human functions, including the way you react to stress. Too little water consumption, for example, induces feelings of lethargy and fatigue, and lowers your resistance to anxiety.

Why? Under stress, your body increases production of red and white cells, and injects increased amounts of clotting agents into the bloodstream; this 'thickened' blood (to use a kitchen-variety metaphor) can contribute to all sorts of conditions from circulatory problems such as heart attack through to feelings of pressure and light-headedness.

Often, an antidote to these conditions is hydration: the intake of water. The simple addition of more water to your diet not only assists in maintaining a feeling of calm, but may also help in the prevention of hypertension, heart ailments, stroke, respiratory problems, constipation, headache, tooth decay, even the aging process itself.

But probably its most visible effect is the way it adds youthfulness, suppleness and even radiance to your skin.

More pertinent to this book, however, water induces calm.

I cannot tell you how much water consumption it takes to relax you in a moment of crisis. I can tell you, however, that several glasses of water, *at room temperature*, will have an immediate effect.

Moreover, if you habitually maintain a reasonable intake, your ability to fight stress, and your resistance to the effects of stress, will be increased. In many cases, *dramatically* increased.

How much water does it take to keep you feeling healthy and calm? An ideal I've seen espoused time and time again is eight full glasses a day.

Many popular cleansing and healing therapies demand considerably more water intake than eight glasses a day. One Chinese water therapy I have heard of demands an intake of one bucketful on rising of a morning – while that may sound excessive, I know several authorities in this area who each consume eight glasses of boiled water on rising every morning of their life, and claim great health advantages as a result.

For our purposes, however, eight glasses a day is a minimum.

To some, that may seem like quite a quantity. I would suggest that it is a minimum! *Because the more water you habitually drink, the more you like to drink and the better you'll feel as a result of it. It's as simple as that.*

Calm waters

For maximum calming effect, water should be drunk at room temperature or *slightly* cooler. Chilled water is not the ideal, although it is preferable to cola, tea or coffee. So if you feel you must drink chilled water for the sake of dietary interest, then go ahead – it is a better alternative than most other beverages.

Even with the best intentions, however, you may have difficulty maintaining interest if the eight glasses you choose to drink come straight from the average tap.

Does this mean you have to buy large quantities of brand-name bottled mineral waters? Not at all.

To my mind, the most satisfying water of them all is the spring water that you see trucks delivering to city offices. I buy it in a large 19-litre (4-gallon) bottle I have delivered to my home. Extravagant? This 'indulgence' costs about the same as three or four bottles of cola, and lasts much, much longer. But there are cheaper and more convenient alternatives.

Add a water purifier to your regular water supply and you have an endless supply of clean, refreshing drinking water. There are many different kinds of purifiers available today – the exotic ones producing water as pure as you could ever hope for, and some of the lower cost versions being available on the supermarket shelves. One particular model I was impressed with was an earthenware type, with a small tap at the bottom. This not only purified the water that was poured into it, but kept the water at a cool, refreshing temperature all year round.

Distilled water is also readily available these days. Because it has no taste, however, you may find it less than interesting. (Newcomers to the wonder of water are often surprised to hear of it described as having 'taste', but most water does. And there is nothing quite so refreshing, nor so satisfying, as a water that suits your taste.)

Some like it hot

This is a secret which, on the surface, may not look like such a breakthrough. Try it a couple of times and I assure you will thank me for it.

What I write of is an alternative to tea and coffee, as well as to cola and fruit juices. Yet it can be as refreshing as any of them.

It costs nothing to buy, yet requires hardly any preparation at all.

But, most important of all, it will help you to relax through the day or before going to bed – especially if you use it as a substitute for tea or coffee.

It's a cup of hot water.

While this may sound dull and uninspiring, you'll find that after the first couple of sips it's not much different to any weak tea or coffee. After a few cups (that is, after you're used to the absence of caffeine), you'll be surprised at just how refreshing it can be. But, if you want to liven it up, simply add a slice of lemon.

CALM WATER

- Drink at least 8 glasses of water a day.
- Drink 2 glasses of water on rising, and one before meals.
- Drink water (2 sips to 1) every time you drink alcohol or coffee.
- Keep a jug or bottle of water at your desk, in your car and at your bedside.
- Drink cool water in preference to soft drinks.
- Drink hot water in preference to tea and coffee.

Calm Herbs and Remedies

Although we have covered the calming properties of many herbal teas, there are other natural remedies worthy of consideration.

According to herbalists, generalised recommendations about herbs are not as efficient as more direct prescriptions, because different herbs work better with different personality types.
Chamomile, for example, is meant to work best for those types who will tell you a whole day's story, noting every minor detail, in a sitting. Skullcap works best for people who exhibit their stress in neck pain and the top of head. Valerian works best for people who show their nervousness, anxiety in physical constraints, entwined fingers, and so on. Even so, I believe that while it may be true that certain herbs work better for certain personality types, they all work to some extent on everybody.

A quality most of them possess is the holistic way in which they function. Not only do these herbs and remedies contain the necessary ingredients to produce calm now, but they also have properties that help the body to heal and cope on an ongoing basis – something pharmaceutical remedies seldom achieve. So important is the study of many age-old herbal therapies becoming, that phytotomy (the dissection and study of plants) and phyto-chemistry (plant chemistry) are now some of the fastest growing disciplines of modern science.

A variety of well-known calm herbs and remedies follow. A visit to the health food store will unearth even more.

Valerian   Often described as 'nature's tranquilliser' because it exerts a powerful sedating action on the central nervous system. It is derived from the dried root of the valerian plant, which is common throughout Europe.

Valerian is available in tablet form (from health food stores and some pharmacies) as well as in powered form for brewing.

As a natural, fast-acting relaxant – one that you can call upon at times of great stress – valerian is without equal. *But, like all powerful sedatives (and stimulants), it should be used with discretion.*

Evening primrose   Has gained a reputation for itself in recent years as a treatment for PMS (pre menstrual syndrome) which is, I believe, an extremely stressful condition. Evening primrose is also an excellent treatment for other stressful conditions.

Even though it comes in the form of an oil, evening primrose is usually purchased in capsules.

However, the usefulness of evening primrose oil extends much farther than PMS. Its main agent, gamma-linolenic acid (GLA), is thought to be effective for the treatment of both hypertension and the lowering of blood pressure.

Hops   Hops have long been known for their sedative qualities. Several modern studies have confirmed what many people throughout Europe have known for centuries – that hops are a great aid to sleep and relaxation.

For maximum effectiveness, you need to get them fresh or at least recently ground. Then, simply add a couple of teaspoons to a litre (2 pints) of boiling water, simmer a few minutes, and leave to sit for half an hour. If necessary, you can sweeten the resultant liquid before drinking.

Skullcap   Another of nature's sedatives. Second in potency only to valerian, it is available in capsule form from health food stores or, if purchased in dried form, can be prepared in a similar way to hops.

Skullcap is also used as a treatment for arthritis and high cholesterol.

Tarragon One of the more popular herbs in French cuisine. The French have known for centuries, though, that this glorious herb has wider applications than culinary.

Steep a teaspoon of common, garden-variety dried tarragon in a litre (2 pints) of hot water for half an hour and the resultant drink is a powerful antidote to insomnia and tension. A small handful of fresh tarragon will produce a similar, but more refreshing, effect.

Catnip One of the mint family of herbs. The relaxing agent in catnip is nepelactone, the chemical structure of which is remarkably similar to the valepotriates that are derived from valerian.

To use catnip, simply add a teaspoon of it to 500 ml (1 pint) of freshly boiled water. For maximum effect, let it steep for 20 minutes before drinking.

You can buy catnip in dried form or in tea bags from health food stores. And, of course, if you ever come across the fresh variety, use that in preference.

Ginseng One of the most revered, most scorned, most mystical, most scoffed-at plants since marijuana, ginseng is rightly known as an exotic herb. It plays a prominent role in Chinese medicine, it is highly prized in areas of Georgia and Russia, it is the basis of a popular Korean soft drink, it comes from a variety of plants and it is extremely rare. This also makes it expensive, and results in a proliferation of counterfeit products. (Also, there is quite a difference between 'ordinary' ginseng and the highly desirable Siberian ginseng.)

> Taken daily over a period of weeks, ginseng is both an aid to stress relief and a counter to the effects of stress on the body. It is renowned for its ability to both stimulate the nervous system and relax it at the same time.

Taken daily over a period of weeks, ginseng is both an aid to stress relief and a counter to the effects of stress on the body. It is renowned for its ability to both stimulate the nervous system and relax it at the same time.

Sound like one of those paradoxical Zen koans?

Be warned, though, ginseng is known most of all as a sexual aid. Millions of satisfied users around the world consider it to be one of nature's most powerful aphrodisiacs. Use it with discretion!

L-tryptophan While not a herb, this is included here as one of the most powerful relaxants I have encountered. It is a manufactured copy of the amino acid tryptophan, which the body produces as an aid to sleep and relaxation. (It is found naturally in meat and milk, which explains why you feel sleepy after eating a steak.) Several years ago, one of the most popular anti-stress remedies available from the health food stores was L-tryptophan. As a treatment of a variety of disorders, especially those relating to stress and insomnia, it was considered to be fast and remarkably effective. However, it was also linked with an illness known as 'eosinophilia-myalgia syndrome' (EMS). And, even though subsequent American studies reportedly traced this to one particular batch imported from Japan, L-tryptophan is no longer available 'over the counter' in many countries, but only on prescription.

Other herbs worthy of consideration include passion flower, wild lettuce, jamaica dogwood, lemon balm, motherwort, rosemary, St John's wort and mistletoe.

Bach remedies

The Bach Flower remedies, developed in the Thirties by Dr Edward Bach, a London bacteriologist and homeopathic physician, have attracted hundreds of thousands of dedicated users over the past half-century.

Applying the theory that the essence of certain flowers can be extracted and utilised to correct a person's psychic balance, and thus put him or her on the path to wellness, the Bach remedies have gained a reputation that is nothing short of amazing. Many prominent people I know swear by their use.

Bach Flower therapy is too specialised an area for me to do any justice in this book. Besides, the fundamentals of its philosophy are the antithesis of what this book is about: instant solutions. Bach remedies and homeopathy are designed to correct subtle physiological imbalances, and to enhance a person's natural healing state – in most cases, this is a long-term project.

Ironically, one of the best known Bach remedies, the Rescue Remedy, is renowned for its immediacy.

Rescue remedy Probably the most popular and commercially well-known of the Bach treatments. It contains rock rose, cherry plum, star of Bethlehem, impatiens and clematis. Whilst not intended for ongoing use, Rescue Remedy is useful for quick relief – providing a pronounced calming effect – from stresses that range from emotional trauma to physical conditions such as burns, strains and abrasions. Some people use it to great effect when confronted by even the smallest, everyday anxieties. It is widely available at health food stores.

Homeopathy

Homeopathy is concerned with the promotion of health through a holistic approach to the constitution. For that very reason, it is impossible for me to single out specific remedies for stress or anxiety. A homeopathic therapist would need to consider the 'big picture' of your state of emotional and physical health before making a recommendation.

The principle behind homeopathy is that by ingesting minute, activated doses of mineral, herbal or even animal toxins you stimulate or activate the body's healing powers. It is based on the same 'law of similars' used in producing many well-known inoculations and antivenenes.

In the search for longer term solutions, homeopathy may be worth closer investigation.

Mineral therapy

Another, lesser-known field of naturopathy is called mineral therapy. It is rather single-minded in its philosophy, espousing the claim that the 'missing link' in the understanding of disease and illness is usually mineral deficiency.

The purpose of mineral therapy, therefore, is to treat these ailments by correcting the body's mineral imbalances – that is, by ingesting specified minerals in the form of tablets or mixtures.

23

CALM AROMAS

Although its name was first coined around 1928, it's one of the oldest therapies in the world, with origins more than 6000 years old. Now it's one of the world's newest 'discoveries'.

This is aromatherapy. Not only are we witnessing a massive surge in popularity for this pleasantly effective phenomenon in 'alternative' marketplaces, but we are also seeing its acceptance in the wider, more conventional community – in the Western world, as well as throughout Asia. Aficionados the world over believe a 30-minute aroma cocktail can relieve the stress and tension of living in a stressful city; people are manufacturing their own healing perfumes; you can buy skilfully scented socks, ties and underwear; and there are even alarm clocks in Japan that wake you with a whiff of pine and eucalyptus.

Aromatherapy was once an ancient Chinese form of herbal medicine, utilising pure, essential plant extracts. Today it is fast becoming recognised as a science, the science of 'aromacology', the study of effects that fragrances have on the way we feel and behave. Research has now shown that certain scents do produce distinct physical effects. Peppermint and lemon, for example, have a stimulating effect on the nervous system (and can actually increase a worker's productivity) while a mix of rosemary and lemon is said to improve concentration.

However it is in the area of relaxation and stress reduction that aromas are believed to be at their most powerful. Indeed, research has shown that the scents of certain essential oils stimulate the production of serotonin in the brain. (Serotonin, you will recall, is the sedative neurochemical that causes slow-wave sleep.)

How an oil becomes essential

Aromatherapy depends on pure essential oils for its power. These oils are derived from a broad range of plants, flowers, bark, seeds, leaves, resins and gums, and are extracted in such minute volumes that it takes more a tonne of flowers, in some instances, to produce 500 ml (1 pint) of oil. This small quantity of pure oil, however, goes a long way – because only a few drops are used on each occasion.

These are not heavy oils such as you will find in the kitchen, but concentrated essences that are not only flammable, but evaporative as well – this is why they are blended with heavier oils for everyday use. So light are they, in fact, that they will begin to penetrate the skin, and take effect, almost instantly they are applied.

For maximum effectiveness, essential oils should be totally pure, and this naturally involves the most stringent testing and analysis in extraction and production.

The calm oils

Essential oils are at their most effective in the treatment of stress and in the encouragement of relaxation.

Scents of vanilla, orange blossom, rose, chamomile and lavender (and other floral fragrances) have a noticeable calming effect on the way you feel, while lavender, sandalwood and nutmeg help you shrug off the ill-effects of stress. Patchouli oil helps eliminate anxiety and lifts the mood (it is also said to be an aphrodisiac, but stressed people don't have to worry about that, do they?).

Lavender is probably the most useful of them all – not only does it help you to relax, but it also eases aches and pains, such as headache. Great-grandmother instinctively knew of these attributes when she carried about a handkerchief perfumed with 'lavender water' or 'rose water'.

The characteristics of calm oils

We can identify a number of oils that have distinct calming properties. Some of these oils share other characteristics as well. For example, basil is a calming oil as well as an 'uplifting' oil (and one to be avoided during pregnancy).

Chamomile, on the other hand, is not classified as an uplifting oil, yet it has useful properties in the treatment of stress and stress conditions.

Consult the chart below for a complete list of these oils and their characteristics.

CALM OILS	UPLIFTING OILS	STRESS OILS	OILS TO AVOID IN PREGNANCY
Basil	Basil		Basil
Bay			Bay
Bergamot	Bergamot		
Cedarwood			
Chamomile		Chamomile	
Cinnamon			
Comfrey			Comfrey
Cypress			
Frankinsense			
Geranium	Geranium	Geranium	
Hyssop			Hyssop
Juniper	Juniper		Juniper
Lavender	Lavender	Lavender	
Marjoram		Marjoram	Marjoram
Melissa	Melissa	Melissa	Melissa
Neroli (orange blossom)			
Patchouli			
		Peppermint	
Rose			
Sage (Clary)			Sage (Clary)
Sandalwood		Sandalwood	
Ylang Ylang			

Useful combinations

For purposes of relaxation and producing a sense of calm, consider *combinations* of the above oils. Experiment with different combinations to determine the effects they produce, taking care never to mix more than three oils.

A particularly attractive combination for me is marjoram, neroli (orange blossom) and bergamot. Another is lavender, bergamot and just a hint of sandalwood (in the ratio of 3:2:1). Experiment and you will be rewarded.

How do you choose the right combinations for you? Easy. Just follow your nose and be guided by what you find pleasant or appealing. Your body will guide you in your choice.

How to use them

A wonderful quality about aromatic oils is the many pleasant ways you can use them – soak in them, smear them over you, inhale them . . .

Following are some of the better known methods of using them. However, I am sure you will think of others if the need to be creative moves you.

NOTE

The quantity of oil I have recommended depends entirely on the quality of the oil you are using. The quality of essential oils you buy over the counter varies greatly: so where you might need only 2 drops of one brand, you might need several of another. Be guided by the labels and the price; then, trust your nose and your instinct – you'll know if you're using too much.

Bathing

This is probably the oldest known way of using aromatic oils. Simply add 10 drops (or more) of your chosen oil or oil mixture to a warm bath, turn down the lights, and immerse yourself in this pleasurable experience. Remember to use Power Breathing as you lie there.

Massage

We have already covered how useful massage can be as a way of soothing the most persistent tensions. By adding 2 per cent (or more) calming essential oils to the oil you use as a massage base (a bland one, such as apricot or jojoba) you can make the experience doubly effective.

Foot baths

Find deep levels of relaxation by adding 4–5 drops of calming oil to a warm foot bath while you practise Power Breathing. Foot massage during this procedure will calm even the most stressed individual.

Vaporisation

There are a variety of devices that allow you to create a calming mood through vaporisation of the oil. These include specially crafted clay vaporisers, ring burners that use the heat from a light bulb, electric humidifiers, even electric 'bubblers'. This is the most popular method of accessing the calming powers of essential oils.

Direct application

The simplest way to access the calming properties of an essential oil is to apply it directly to your body. Add the lightest smear to your pulse points and wear it as a perfume. Alternatively, mix a few drops with distilled water to make a 'cologne', or add 1 per cent essential oil to a carrier oil as a facial oil, or 3–4 per cent to a carrier oil as a body lotion.

Compress

Although the mention of compresses may have unpleasant medical connotations, this method is one of the easiest ways to use essential oils. Simply soak a clean cotton cloth in a cup of warm water with 5–10 drops of oil added. Wring out, and lay across the forehead area as you perform Power Breathing exercises.

Inhalation

Add 4–12 drops to a bowl of steaming water, place a towel over your head and breathe deeply and slowly. Use only in extreme cases of stress and anxiety.

Others

- Add a few drops to wood an hour before lighting a fire.
- Use scented wax candles.
- Add a few drops to your pillow or your handkerchief.
- Use calming essential oils in conjunction with any of the other techniques in this book.

Although incense is not usually considered in the same forums as essential oils, it, too, works on the psycho-neuro centre of the brain and stimulates the production of serotonin, which induces calm.

AROMATIC PLUNGE

- Run a warm bath, not too hot.
- Add 5–10 drops (or more) of your chosen calm oil, or mixture of oils. Close doors and windows so the calming aromas remain in the room.
- Slowly immerse yourself in the warm water, deeply breathing the aromas.
- Commence Power Breathing while you lie there and relax.

D.I.Y. OILS

- ■ Add a litre (2 pints) of boiling water to a cup of flower buds or leaves, according to your preference.
- ■ Allow to cool.
- ■ Strain the liquid and add it to your warm bath water.
- ■ In a quiet, darkened bathroom, immerse yourself in this soothing cocktail.
- ■ Commence Power Breathing while you lie there and relax.

24

BREAKING PATTERNS

One of the overriding principles of *Instant Calm* is that the harmful effects of negative stress can be overcome simply by reversing the physical, emotional or physiological symptoms that cause it.

If you know that a physical pattern of clenched teeth and tight jaw muscles increases the stress levels in your body, then you reverse that pattern to decrease the stress – you slacken the jaw muscles. Many of these physical 'reversing' techniques have already been covered in other sections.

> If you know that a physical pattern of clenched teeth and tight jaw muscles increases the stress levels in your body, then you reverse that pattern to decrease the stress – simply slacken the jaw muscles.
> If you know that a pattern of negative thinking increases your propensity to stress-related discomfort, then you reverse that pattern to decrease the stress – you employ positive-thinking techniques.

But what if your stress is caused by your attitudes? Or your lifestyle?

The following chapter highlights a number of the more common high-stress attitudinal and lifestyle issues. (Not surprisingly, you will find many of them fall into that Type A behavioural pattern, which is covered in greater detail later in this book.) Accompanying these are the reverses – the frames of mind you would adopt if you were to have low-stress attitudes or lifestyle.

As an example: if you know that an emotional pattern of negative thinking increases your propensity to stress-related discomfort, then you reverse that pattern to decrease the stress – you employ positive-thinking techniques.

Whatever the remedy, you will often find that simply being able to see your problem in its proper perspective means you are a long way down the track towards solving it.

Reverse Lifestyle and Attitudinal Patterns

THE HIGH-STRESS ATTITUDE

You suffer ongoing feelings of boredom, anxiety and helplessness.

You see no relief from the ever-present anxieties and pressures of life.

You feel you always are the victim and that you're heading nowhere.

There's so much you have to do, so little time to do it.

You wonder if you will ever get on top of things.

You just can't escape the feeling that something's going to go wrong.

You're never able to relax and have a good time.

You feel guilty about not doing something 'worthwhile' at all times.

Life is so terribly, terribly serious.

THE LOW-STRESS ATTITUDE

Your life is varied – quieter times, interspersed with periods of stimulating, challenging activities.

You are disciplined about setting aside regular 'alone time' – where your only objective is detachment and relaxation.

You do an honest audit of your strengths and weaknesses, then concentrate on your strengths.

You take the time to define your goals and are realistic about the expectations you set for yourself.

You accept only achievable tasks and deadlines, renegotiating either if necessary.

You've taken a cold, hard look at what could go wrong, assessed its likelihood, then taken positive steps to reduce the possibility or to dismiss it as unlikely.

You appreciate that just having fun is an end in itself. After all, having fun is half the fun.

You acknowledge that 'meaningless', playful activities are an essential part of a well-balanced life.

You know that life has its light and amusing side – even for busy and successful people. You can even laugh at yourself at times.

THE HIGH-STRESS ATTITUDE

Because of who you are, everyone expects you to think or perform in a certain way.

Your work is always such a drudge – unfulfilling, unrewarding and dull.

Whether through conflict, jealousy or inertia, your relationships are a regular source of pain and frustration.

Life's a bitch, but you suffer in silence.

You'll never be able to give up smoking, drinking, or eating to excess.

You feel there is no point in struggling, as the misfortunes of life are inevitable.

THE LOW-STRESS ATTITUDE

You acknowledge that great things usually come from individuals – as opposed to role players.

You immerse yourself in everything you do – totally and wholeheartedly.

You treat relationships as a creative process based on independence and individuality. Naturally, you choose your friends on this basis.

You learn and employ assertiveness skills to get what you want from life.

You embrace the benefits of an active, moderate and healthy lifestyle (which, in turn, usually means you will discard those excesses).

You have choice in everything you do. You constantly reassure yourself: *I am in control of my own destiny.*

The Calm Slowdown

Some of the more noticeable patterns of a person in an advanced state of stress relate to speed.

Conversation is speeded up. Words come at machine-gun pace. Such is the urge to get communication out of the way as rapidly as possible that, in one extreme instance I know of, a man articulates only every second or third word as he reads something to you. Take ... word ... is ... pain ... the ...

> Just as you can quieten a distressed child by speaking softly, just as you can appease an angry adult by breathing easily, speaking slowly and appearing totally calm, just as you can soothe a hysterical person by speaking in slow, measured tones, so, too, you can calm yourself by adopting these outward expressions.

Another pattern you cannot help noticing is the fidgeting: wringing hands, drumming or fiddling fingers, shuffling feet, tugging collars, crossing and uncrossing legs. In more extreme cases, you will see trembling hands and grinding teeth as well.

The final area of noticeability is the breathing. A stressed, nervous person breathes in shallow, rapid breaths. Sometimes, he or she may even experience breathing difficulties such as shortage of breath or hyperventilation.

The patterns of a calm, relaxed person are the opposite.

His/her breathing is slow and deep. His/her speech rhythms are slow and relaxed. His/her mannerisms as well as hand and feet movements are languid – almost lazy.

Could it be that, just by adopting the superficial characteristics of a calm person, you can actually reverse the stressful feelings that caused you to fidget and speak rapidly in the first place? Of course you can.

Just as you can quieten a distressed child by speaking softly, just as you can appease an angry adult by breathing easily, speaking slowly and appearing totally calm, just as you can soothe a hysterical person by speaking in slow, measured tones, so, too, you can calm yourself by adopting these outward expressions.

(You will also be aware of the reverse of this: how easy it is for one anxious individual to spread a feeling of unease throughout a group, and how easy it is to make someone else angry simply by adopting an angry attitude when you are near them.)

The technique

The Calm Slowdown works because of the *physical* actions that you take to overcome an anxious or highly stressed state. These actions are designed to be the opposite of those you exhibit while stressed – even if you are not conscious of doing so.

The first, and most important, step is to get your breathing into order. Spend a minute or so using the Power Breathing technique until your breathing pattern is deep and slow. (If you do this correctly, it will seem unnaturally slow to you at first; but persist, and you will soon feel comfortable with the rhythm.)

The next step is to make a conscious effort to slow down all of your physical actions. Speak slower – even slower than you think sounds natural. Every time you move your feet and your hands, force them to move slower and more purposefully. Think about every movement you make. Avoid the *superficial* characteristics of a stressed person: folding your arms, crossing and uncrossing your legs, twitching, scratching and so on. Every moment you make should be slow and purposeful. Think about it. Slow and purposeful. *Even slower than you think seems natural.*

If need be, you can perform the Calm Exercises on pages 73–5, knowing that these will force you to slow down.

As well as all of the above, consider slowing *everything* down.

Walk slower.

Drive slower.

Think slower.

THE CALM SLOWDOWN

- Remember the Conditions of Calm.
- Commence Power Breathing techniques. Concentrate on making your breathing slower and deeper. Do this for a minute or so.
- Make a conscious effort to slow down all of your physical actions.
- Force your feet and hands to move slowly and purposefully. Think about every movement you make. Avoid folding your arms, crossing and uncrossing your legs, twitching and so on. Every moment should be slow and purposeful. *Even slower than you believe seems natural.*
- Make a conscious effort to slow down your speech. Think about the pace of your words. *Speak slower than you think sounds natural.*
- Even if the pace seems unnatural to you, continue to breathe, move and speak slowly and purposefully, thinking about every physical action you make. Continue to do this even *after* you are feeling calm and relaxed, and you will remain that way.

Change of Face

The facial muscles are the site of so much of the tension you carry about with you. Not only do they influence the way you feel, but they also communicate these feelings to the world – there is no mistaking the demeanour of the anxious or stressed person: the frown, the tight lips, the clenched jaw.

It is so easy to reverse these facial characteristics, thus beginning to reverse the way you feel.

We covered the major musculature changes earlier in the Calm Demeanour on page 130. One of these changes is simply extraordinary in its potential, yet so basic in application that is liable to be overlooked.

It's a pattern-reversing technique that you've been using since childhood. It provides maximum relief to tense facial muscles. It is the 'normal' muscular position for most relaxed human faces. It has an inherent meaning, and is accompanied by a certain attitude that everyone feels comfortable with and takes delight in.

It is a smile.

A smile is the reverse of the tense facial pattern described above. Better still, a smile is the perfect 'Programmed Conditioned Response' that we investigated in the Calm Touch on page 115. According to recent research, there is a definite correlation between a certain type of smile (the 'wrinkly eye' variety) and feeling good. In fact, this kind of smile produces an instant neurological stimulation of the pleasure centre of your brain.

Take this smile a bit further, into a laugh, and the benefits are multiplied many times. The act of laughing not only makes you feel better, but has direct physiological benefits such as helping to stabilise the blood pressure and to assist circulation. This is no doubt why laughter has been described as 'aerobics for the inside'.

How do you do it? Very funny.

CHANGE OF FACE

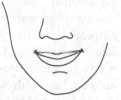

- Remain on the lookout for things that make you laugh.
- If nothing makes you laugh, pretend you find something amusing. Or appealing. And smile.

Another face

Go on, admit it: you take yourself too seriously.

You should not feel alarmed: this condition is common to most worriers and is central to the Type A stereotype. Saying 'don't take yourself too seriously' has no effect because it is, in itself, a serious suggestion.

Many years ago I was introduced to a course called Clowning. Its purpose was to release people from their own pomposity and seriousness, to teach them a new fun way of looking at life. The course was relatively straightforward: you were taught how to apply clown makeup, how to dress like a clown and how to act like a clown; then you were expected to perform. Oddly enough, it worked. Those who attended learned a whole new batch of skills that enabled them to dispense with their seriousness, and become more relaxed and comfortable with themselves.

Here is a simpler way.

Take yourself along to one of those enclosed photo booths. Ensure no one else is about, then draw the curtains. Insert your coins. Take a deep breath.

Now, pull four of the most ridiculous faces you are capable of. It is impossible to be too ridiculous in this exercise, go to the maddest imaginable extremes. Do whatever comes unnaturally. Let yourself go. Try to embarrass yourself.

You will now have four photographs that can change the way you look at yourself – in an instant. When you find yourself feeling unnecessarily serious (that is, when you're feeling tense, stressed and carrying the weight of the world on your shoulders), simply whip out these photos and let those ridiculous faces do the rest.

If you're a serious type of person you'll probably say such a technique would not work for you. But if you're that serious, it will work for you best of all.

Seriously.

Walk Calm

Ah, how we love to overlook the obvious. What is the one thing you tend to do when you reach the peak of anxiety, when your world is collapsing about you, when your pulse is racing and you believe you just can't cope a moment longer? You begin to pace.

Could it be that your subconscious knows something your conscious mind does not? Of course it does. It knows that walking is one of nature's great antidotes to stress, a sure way of dealing with those 'stress chemicals' that are produced in fight or flight situations.

This is why I am such a great advocate of this activity.

When stress levels rise, drop what you're doing and take a walk. When anxiety levels increase, walk away from them. When your problems get you down, get up and walk them off.

Walk around the block. Better still, walk in a park. Walk with your back straight, head high, shoulders back. Imagine you are taller than you are. Look people in the eye, not with a challenge but with pride.

Walk for 30 minutes. Even better, walk for an hour. Briskly, so your pulse rate is increased and there is a film of sweat on your brow.

If you devote the time, there is no better exercise for the elimination of stress and for your overall wellbeing.

WALK CALM

- Whenever you feel under pressure or suffering from anxiety, take to the street.
- Walk briskly – shoulders back, head held high.
- Imagine you are taller than you are. Look people in the eye.
- Continue walking until your pulse rate rises and there is a film of sweat on your brow.

A Calm Place

An unusual characteristic of people suffering the long-term effects of stress is the way their problems become associated with particular places and behaviours.

The stressed-out executive, for example, suffers most when he sits at his desk. As these stress levels continue and become habitual, sitting at that desk becomes associated – certainly on a subconscious level – with feelings of stress; all that executive has to do is sit at that particular desk and tensions or anxiety will surface.

This kind of association is simply a negative example of the Programmed Condition Response (PCR) we outlined earlier: you establish a pattern of stressful behaviour or thinking, and a stressful reaction is triggered whenever you repeat that behaviour.

So how are you meant to cope with these negative PCR-associated situations? Avoid them altogether? Stay home from work? Change offices? Not sit at your desk?

The solution utilises the same mechanism that caused the problem in the first place – a programmed condition response. A *positive* programmed condition response.

For example: if most of your stressful associations at work arise in one particular office chair, you simply create another place where your associations are the reverse of this – where you feel calm, relaxed and powerful. You might nominate another chair in your office for this purpose. This then becomes a refuge, a Calm Place you can visit or move to whenever the need arises.

But before it becomes a Calm Place, certain conditioning has to take place.

When you're feeling relaxed and light-hearted, which most people seem to manage for at least a few minutes in the average day, move to this chair. Savour the feelings while sitting there. Build the association with feeling good while you're in that place. (To ensure this happens even faster, refer to the Calm Touch on page 115.) Then, whenever you feel tense or under pressure, all you have to do is move to this Calm Place to break the pattern. For maximum effectiveness, you may choose to employ other techniques from this book while you're sitting there; not only will they add to the effectiveness but, in time, will become unnecessary – as the positive associations are established.

As simplistic as it may appear, this works like a charm. Several years ago we used a similar technique – to combat writer's block – in an advertising agency I worked for. When the artists and copywriters were stuck for an idea, they would simply move from their regular workplaces to other designated 'creative spaces' until the ideas started flowing again.

Finding relief from stress and tension can work in the same way. So simple, so easy, yet so effective.

A CALM PLACE

- Nominate a specific place where you intend to establish only calm and peaceful feelings. Establish it near any place you regularly feel stressed and under pressure.
- For a week or so, move to this place whenever you're feeling calm and relaxed. Each time you do it, make a point of savouring the pleasure of feeling that way. Alternatively, use the Calm Touch to physically make the association with this Calm Place.
- Then, whenever you feel tense or under pressure, move to this place.
- If simply moving there is not sufficient to overcome all feelings of tension or anxiety, use other techniques from this book while you are there.
- Use Power Breathing as well.

Physical Disconnection

Have you ever noticed how tense people seem to thrive on tense situations? The more uncomfortable they feel in a particular situation, the more likely they are to remain in that situation until their discomfort gets out of hand.

> 'I feel so miserable standing out here in the cold.'
> 'Then get out of the cold.'

Whether we are conscious of it or not, we are guilty of such seemingly irrational behaviour more often than we would care to admit. Even though there is nothing we can do about it, we continue to worry about the effects of a decision that has already been made. Even though we know there will be no resolution, we continue to engage others in futile argument. Even though we know it increases our tension levels, we continue to tell ourselves we need a coffee, cigarette, drink or television to relax. Even though we know our stress levels are rising, we continue to sweat over those taxation figures, and sweat over those figures, and sweat over those figures . . .

If this is not the product of masochism or a desire for self-destruction, then it may be a simple inability to recognise stressful situations as they arise. More often, though, it is the result of stressed people being driven by an inexplicable need to triumph over the situations that bind them. And this is seldom achieved.

So the first step in solving your problem is to acknowledge that you are not going to solve your problem every time. At least, not at that particular moment. Having acknowledged this, you can then go about easing your stress.

Whenever you find yourself in a highly stressed state, physically move away from the stressor. *Physically* move. And do this in a way that is physically different to the way you'd normally do it.

After you have made a *physical* disconnection from your stressor, it is time to concentrate on making the most of your disconnection. For whatever time you're involved in this diversionary activity, totally immerse yourself in the experience. Savour the sights and sounds, observe the people who are nearby, take note of environmental differences to what you've come from. Take *pleasure* in these differences.

What if you become tense and anxious in a situation you cannot walk away from?

PHYSICAL DISCONNECTION

- When you find yourself in a highly stressed state, move away from the place where you're suffering. Physically move.
- Do so in a way that is physically different to the way you'd normally do it. If you'd normally sit down, go for a walk. If you'd normally watch television, take a bus into the city to see a movie.
- Totally immerse yourself in the new experience. Savour the sights and sounds, observe the people, take note of environmental differences. Take pleasure in the differences.
- If you cannot move, physically change the way you address your stressful situation. Change the way you sit, the way you're dressed, the chair you occupy, or the tools you use, for a few hours.
- Use Power Breathing and other techniques from this book.

A physical disconnection does not have to involve changes of location. As an alternative, you can physically change the way you address the situation that bothers you.

> If you become tense and anxious at work, instead of sitting at your desk with a cup of coffee, take a brisk walk around the block. If you become tense and anxious at home, instead of sitting down and turning on the radio, take a bus into the city to see a movie. If that's what you'd normally do, take a train across town to see an art show, or cycle to a neighbouring suburb to see a garden display.

If, for example, you're feeling anxious yet cannot leave the telephone switchboard, do something physically different while you operate it: remove an item of underwear (subtly, now) so you can work there feeling free and daring; take off your shoes and rest your bare feet on a telephone directory; swap chairs or keyboards with a co-worker for a few hours.

And, just as you would if you'd moved to another location, totally immerse yourself in the differences involved in these changes or new experiences.

25

DEALING WITH SPECIFIC FEARS AND ANXIETIES

If you suffer from specific fears and anxieties – be they real, imagined, reasonable or absurd – you can be thankful. For you have an advantage that most worriers do not.

Pity instead those who suffer from *non-specific* fears and anxieties – they're not sure why they feel tense or anxious, they just feel tense and anxious; and they become even more tense and anxious trying to identify the source of their tensions.

If you are a person of this type, worry becomes a self-fuelling condition, and the fact that you worry about one thing is sufficient reason for you to begin worrying about others. The pattern continues until you do something to break it.

Much of *Instant Calm* is dedicated to breaking these patterns. This chapter, however, is dedicated to dealing with the *specific* worries and anxieties that bother people.

The first and most sensible way of dealing with these is to approach the problem in the same way you would approach any work task or chore:

- identify your problem
- determine the outcome you want to achieve in relation to it
- weigh up the positives and negatives of the various courses of action

- take the steps necessary to achieving your outcome
- say goodbye to the problem (or try another course).

Sounds easy, doesn't it? But, the subconscious being what it is, this logical, commonsense approach will end in frustration – because the subconscious needs to be *charmed* into doing what you want. Following are a few techniques that will work for you in this way.

The Framing Technique

The Framing Technique we covered on page 104 was conceived to transport you from the stressed state into a calm state. However, it is also an excellent technique for dealing with specific fears and anxieties. If you can visualise these – usually all it takes is a little imagination and applied creativity – you can deal with them in this way.

Say you're afraid of an irate neighbour. With the Framing Technique, all you have to do is conjure up a picture of this angry person, fuming and puffing. Then, reduce this mental picture until he fits neatly inside a cute little picture frame. Now dress him up in an amusing costume – a Little Red Riding Hood cape, or high heels and suspenders. Then see how easy it is to deal with him.

Read back over the Framing Technique, and see how it can apply in this case.

Alternative Pretend

The Let's Pretend Technique covered on page 112 was originally conceived for dealing with generalised (that is, non-specific) feelings of tension and anxiety. If, however, your stress is the product of *specific* fears or anxieties, and you feel that these need to be addressed before you can start to feel calm, then they can be treated with this slightly modified technique.

Remember the object of this is to appeal to your subconscious, the place where most fears and anxieties emanate!

Once again, this is a visualisation technique. It requires you to visualise, on your 'big screen', the cause of your anxiety.

Say, for example, your concern is public speaking and you have an important speech coming up. In the first instance, you have to visualise what the speaking venue is going to be like – the stage, the placement of the podium, the size of the audience, the people who will be in attendance, the sounds of coughing and moving chairs in the auditorium. Do not try to visualise yourself in this environment; just the environment itself.

Next comes the pretend stage.

Just pretending now, conjure up a picture of yourself as one of the country's most compelling and confident speakers. People would come from all over the country to hear such a speaker. (If you find this difficult, you may have to model your pretend-self on some other speaker you've seen or know about.)

Imagine how this pretend image of yourself – one of the most sought-after speakers in the country – would approach this speaking engagement.

Imagine how you'd get ready for it. You'd be taking your own

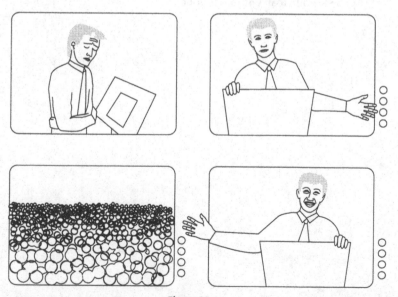

Figure 72

clothes, from your own wardrobe, in your own home. No sign of butterflies or apprehension about what's ahead of you.

You'd be driving there in your own car. Relaxed, confident about how you know your speech will turn out. When you arrived at the location, the doorman would be suitably deferential towards you.

Then you stride out onto that stage, confident as only a great speaker who knows his topic can be. And you speak with the confidence and authority that only a great speaker can summon.

In this exercise you should 'see' the audience, 'hear' their murmurs of agreement, 'feel' what it is like to stand on that stage.

When that pretend image of yourself is firmly in your mind, pretend you can hear the applause. Pretend you can feel the pride in accepting that applause.

Now, 'turn up' the picture, 'turn up' the sound. Wait . . . and absorb what it feels like to be in that confident situation.

When it becomes time for you to stand up and speak in front of a real audience, all you have to do is start Power Breathing and pretend you are that speaker again. And, more importantly, pretend that others see you as that speaker.

Surprise – your fear will have gone!

ALTERNATIVE PRETEND TECHNIQUE

- Remember the Conditions of Calm.
- On your 'big screen', conjure up an image of the place or situation where your fear or anxiety is most likely to occur. Note the colours, the environment, the sounds, the textures.
- Now, *just pretending*, imagine yourself as someone who is totally unfazed by that situation – someone who is confident and in control, and who is known for being unfazed by such things. Picture yourself preparing to place yourself in that situation. Picture yourself getting dressed for the event, driving there in your car.
- Now picture your *pretend-self* approaching that situation. You're calm, confident and totally in control.
- Picture your *pretend-self* handling that situation with aplomb. 'Hear' the sounds, 'feel' the temperature and textures, 'see' what you would be seeing there.
- Next time you really approach such a situation, simply start Power Breathing and pretend you are that person. And, most importantly, pretend that others see you as you are pretending to be.

The Notebook Technique

Many worriers have a dislike for this particular technique, not because it works so elegantly, but because it stabs at the heart of their worries and concerns.

You may think that should be little cause for alarm. But if you accept that most worriers believe their anxieties to be of real significance – if not to the world, then certainly to them – then the Notebook Technique conceals a very real threat.

Because this technique turns worries and anxieties into non-events. It exposes them for the shams that they so often are.

The Notebook Technique is based on the understanding that most people's worries centre on what may happen (or what has already happened). In others words, most stress is caused by expectation – not by the actual event or even the threat of the event, but simply the expectation that the event will happen – or regret.

When scrutinised critically, most concerns of the 'expectation' type are unfounded. Similarly, all concerns about the past are meaningless (unless, of course, they're going to have real repercussions in the future).

The tools you need for this technique are probably already in your possession: a notebook and a pencil. There are two ways of putting them to use.

Short-term worries

> Learn to trust your subconscious in these matters. It will find the solution for you.

The first is a way of dealing with short-term worries – the type that crop up during the day or, in the case of hard-core worriers, in the early hours of the morning.

When these occur, simply get out of bed, write down your problem, then inform yourself that you will deal with the issue at a specific time in the future, say the following day at noon.

Turn making that appointment with yourself into a ritual.

In doing this, not only do you postpone the worry to a time that *you* dictate, but you are well down the track towards finding a solution for it.

If a solution is required, your subconscious will do all the work for you *before* the appointment time. While it is searching for the solution, you can go about life as usual.

Learn to trust your subconscious in these matters. It is infinitely more creative than your conscious mind, and specialises in finding solutions to difficult problems. And all you have to do to ensure it achieves its potential is to place your faith in it, and not use your conscious mind (that is, thinking) to search for the solution.

Please don't underestimate the power of your subconscious performing these tasks. If there is one thing I have learned in the past decade of research into calm, it is to respect the awesomeness of the subconscious.

Trust in yours and it will work for you.

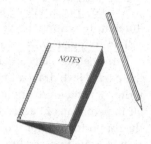

Figure 73a

Figure 73b

More worrying concerns

The second aspect of the Notebook Technique is a way of dealing with concerns that are impossible to get off your mind. (And, therefore, are impossible to turn over to your subconscious for solutions.) It follows a very simple formula.

Take up your pencil and, at the bottom of the page, write your worry (Figure 73b).

'I'm worried about keeping my job.'

'I think my boyfriend might be cheating on me.'

'I am not very popular with women.'

Now, at the top of the page write the outcome you seek when this worry is

Figure 73c

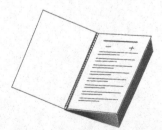

Figure 73d

removed. Ensure that it is worded positively and (according to your situation) realistically. Underline the outcome.

'I will have a long-lasting tenure in my job.'

'My boyfriend will be someone who does not cheat.' (Note this is different to writing 'I will discover my boyfriend is not cheating'.)

'I am popular with women.'

Turn the page. Once again, write the outcome you seek at the top of the page. Next, draw a line down the middle of that page. On the left write '−', and on the right write '+' (Figure 73c). Now, on the left, list all impediments to achieving your outcome. And on the right, list all the opportunities or possibilities that exist (or what qualities or resources you possess) to enable the outcome written at the top of the page.

Turn the page and, once again, write the outcome you seek at the top.

Now list all the ways you can use your qualities and resources in '+' to overcome all the impediments in '−' (Figure 73d). If there are not enough of these qualities and resources, go back a page and add some of the ones you've overlooked.

By the end of that page, two things should have happened: either your worries should now be in perspective and minimised, or a solution achieving your outcome should be staring you in the face.

If for some reason you do not realise these objectives at the end of the process, it may be worth reviewing the outcome you'd written at the top of your page in the first place.

Not only is this technique a useful way of dispensing with worries, it is also one of the most powerful problem-solving techniques that can be used in business. Put it to good use.

THE NOTEBOOK TECHNIQUE

- At the bottom of the page write your major worry.
- At the top of the page write the outcome you seek.
- Turn the page. Once again, write your outcome at the top.
- Divide the page into '−' and '+' columns.
  On the '−' side, write the impediments to achieving your outcome; on the '+', write the qualities and resources you possess that will enable it to happen.
- Turn the page. Once again, write your outcome at the top.
- Now list all the ways you can use your qualities and resources ('+') to overcome the impediments ('−'). If you need more qualities and resources, go back and think up more.
- The end of your worries and a path for achieving your outcome should be on that page.

LONGER-TERM CALM SOLUTIONS

26

LONGER-TERM SOLUTIONS

Now we get serious.

This is the part where we finally acknowledge that, attractive though they may appear, quick fixes are not the ideal long-term solution to stress- and anxiety-related problems. These types of problems usually require significant shifts in lifestyle and attitude.

Those of you who have read my earlier book on this subject, *the Calm Technique*, will know the shifts to which I refer. I assume you have not read it and adopted its principles; if you had, you will have little need for a book called *Instant Calm*.

Assuming, therefore, that you are a newcomer to this topic, let me put to rest any suggestion that I am writing about a difficult, esoteric study. Or that I am writing about some strange form of mystical or spiritual development.

I am writing about a series of simple, enjoyable exercises and principles that can change your life.

Building Blocks of Calm

To become calm, to find real peace and contentment, it is necessary to pay attention to several different aspects of life. I call these the Building Blocks of Calm. They are: commitment, the Calm Technique, diet, exercise, selflessness and attitude.

If we assume you are committed, all you have to do is concentrate on *any three of the following areas.* Ideally, of course, you will concentrate on all of them.

Commitment

The most important consideration in finding long-term calm is commitment. If you acknowledge that a propensity to stress and anxiety is seldom a fleeting condition, and if you are committed to finding a solution to this, you are halfway there.

In the pages that follow, you will find a number of techniques and lifestyle modifications with the power to transform a tense, stress-ridden person into a shining example of calm.

Follow them and you will be tranquil, contented and more able to cope than you would ever have believed possible. Follow them and your life will be enriched beyond all expectations. Follow them and, in years to come, you will look back on this very paragraph as a turning point in your life.

The Calm Technique

The Calm Technique is a simple meditation technique that was covered in great detail in my book of the same title. It, or any other form of meditation, is essential for a happy, well-balanced, healthy way of life.

Every time I write or speak of the powers of meditation, I expose myself to the criticism of over-promising or allowing my enthusiasm to cloud my modesty. Yet the volume of letters I receive, and the number of endorsements and recommendations the Calm Technique has received over the years, continue to confirm my faith in this powerful skill. It is no exaggeration to report that, of all the hundreds of articles and reviews it has attracted throughout the world, there has not been a single criticism of substance.

This has little to do with new thinking or new discoveries. The things I refer to are simple truths and techniques which a large proportion of the world considers commonplace.

If you approach these techniques with dedication and sincerity, if you do not come with intentions of quick fixes or cosmic thrill-seeking, you will discover the life-transforming powers that a real sense of calm can deliver.

(The Calm Technique is covered in greater depth towards the end of this book.)

Diet

If there's one thing that affects your state of mind as much as your health, it's your diet.

As we have discussed in an earlier chapter, certain foods can be described as 'calm foods' and can have a soothing effect on your stress levels – especially in the long term.

■ Concentrate on maintaining an 80:20 balance between the acid-forming foods (wholegrain flour and cereals, fruits, vegetables, especially uncooked), and alkaline-forming foods (coffee, meat, sugar, processed foods, white flour, nuts, preservatives).
■ Eat less (for most people).
■ Eat more vegetables, fruits, complex carbohydrates and whole grains.

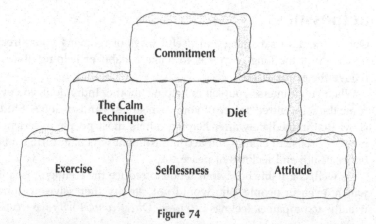

Figure 74

- Eat less fats.
- Ensure your diet is high in vitamins A, C, E and B.
- Drink more water.
- Wherever possible, start your day with fresh fruit or fruit juice, and begin each meal with raw vegetables or a salad. Use fruit or whole-grain bread as snack foods.
- Limit or avoid altogether: coffee, soft drinks, sugar, refined foods, preserved foods and fat-laden snack foods.

Exercise

The importance of exercise to your state of health requires no further discussion here. But exercise is not only good for your body, it is equally as important to your state of mind.

Regular exercise diminishes the effects of stress on the body.

Regular exercise helps you to cope better.

Regular exercise will make you feel more calm and contented.

If the thought of all that stretching and sweating bothers you, take up walking. Not only does walking require no special skills or equipment, it is the most relaxing and one of the most beneficial of all exercises.

There is no better start to a calm day than a brisk, 40-minute walk as the sun rises. Walk. And remember your Power Breathing.

Selflessness

One of the most satisfying and useful ways of relieving your stress – especially in the long term – is to make a habit of helping others to relieve theirs.

When you immerse yourself in helping another individual, you over-come the self-centred nature of your own stresses and anxieties. Studies show that immediately after helping others most people experience a powerful sense of elation and accomplishment which, in turn, leads to better health and feelings of peace.

As well, charitable behaviour tends to reduce the feeling of isolation which, even in people who would not classify themselves as lonely, usually accompanies feelings of stress. *Direct contact with the recipient, however, is a necessary part of the process*; a simple donation may not be sufficient.

For a long-term sense of calm and fulfilment, seek out opportunities to help others. Your efforts will be rewarded.

Attitude

Which comes first: a sense of calm, or a positive, happy outlook on life?

It hardly matters. If you can maintain a state of real calm, you will be positive and happy. Conversely, if you are positive and happy, you will find it easy to be calm.

Optimism is the most important attitude you can pursue. Not only will it help you to be calm, but it will bring increased happiness, better health, more effective relationships and vastly improved communications.

How do you achieve it?

Listen to your conversation and your thoughts. Steer well clear of all negative expressions; strive to find the positive in all you say and think about. When you do succumb to the negative, try bombarding it with positive interpretations of the same thought. Instead of 'I've got so much work to do', try, 'I'm so fortunate to be fully occupied', or, 'It's so rewarding to have useful work and challenges'.

Picture yourself with a smile and boundless enthusiasm. Refer back to that mental picture time and time again throughout the day. Look for every opportunity to laugh.

Finally, throw yourself into every activity you encounter. Even if the task is an unpleasant one, perform it as thoroughly and as conscientiously as is you possibly can. As the students of Zen will tell you, this is one of the most well-established paths to peace and contentment.

27

WORK AND BE CALM

Most of the techniques in this book are as suited to the factory floor as they are to the busy office as they are to the home. Maybe you'll need to apply a little imagination here and there to make them work for you in all situations, but they will work if you make the effort.

The true test of any calm person is when he or she goes to work. It seem that, somehow, those eight or ten hours a day have been specially designed to remove any semblance of calm from your life and, by the end of the day, to burden you with so many pressures and responsibilities that your next day will be exactly the same.

Is that how work seems to you?

To cover all the stresses and anxieties specific to the workplace would take many volumes. And I'm sure at the end of that exercise you'd still find I'd only just scratched the surface.

The causes of workplace stress

Generally, most stress in the workplace occurs as the result of one of four factors: Time, Expectation, Situation, Social. Stressors from each of these areas can be can be addressed by many of the techniques contained within this book.

The one category I have not bothered to cover in great detail is the last, Social, which obviously involves a multitude of relationship factors that no book of techniques could satisfactorily address.

Time

These are the pressures we know best of all. 'Time is money.' Approaching deadlines, time running out, not enough hours in the day. All of these problems can be overcome through attitude, primarily, and sensible time management thereafter.

Expectation

We have covered this elsewhere – anxiety about imagined impending problems or situations. This could involve financial risk, risk of injury, accountability, or more abstract anxieties such as fear of authority and fear of failure.

Situation

This relates to the physical aspects of your employment – position, status, work environment, the amount of control you have over your destiny.

It also relates to environmental factors such as heat, cold, humidity, darkness, glare, dryness, wetness, noise, vibration, pollution (smoke, odours, gases, dust, poisons), dangerous work and physical injury.

Social

Obviously, this deals with the people you work with and work for, how you relate to them and how they relate to you. It may also involve customers and remote sources such as the board or regulatory authorities.

The workplace

A stress-management consultant would, more often than not, strive to solve your stress problems at work by modifying the procedures at your workplace. He or she would probably recommend a range of solutions – from establishing semi-autonomous work groups, to goal-setting exercises, to organisational change. He or she would argue such things as: you should participate in decision-making; you should

Keys to a Stress-free Workplace

The keys to eliminating stress in the workplace – or at least keeping it under control – are almost identical to the keys to being an effective worker. Not surprisingly, they cover each of the most common categories of workplace stress: Time, Expectation, Situation and Social.

TIME

- **Only take on what you know you can do.**
This applies to the responsibilities you accept as much as it does to deadlines. Concentrate on tasks, set reasonable deadlines for yourself, and time takes care of itself.

- **Put aside 20 minutes a day for decision-making and organisation.**
Use this time to plan your day, to tidy your desk, to arrange your tools, to set your objectives. Allow yourself no other thoughts or interruptions. (If your position does not allow you to do this, start work 20 minutes earlier.)

- **Work only one day at a time.**
Work to your maximum during working hours, then leave it all behind when you go home. You can easily pick up where you left off the next day.

EXPECTATION

- **Attempt to control only what's possible for you to control.**
Use the Notebook Technique (page 270) to set out strategies and differentiate between what is achievable and what is not. Then devote your energies only to those tasks you can achieve; hand over the others to someone else.

SITUATION

■ **Appreciate the routine.**

Every job has its routine bits. Learn to use these 'remote control' tasks as stress breaks. Apply the principles from the next section The Total Effort to use these moments fully.

■ **Spend some time not being a cog.**

This could be the most important principle on this page. Spend up to half an hour a day not being a cog in the machine. Take a walk around the block. Have a nap under the desk. Deliver the mail to the post office. This is essential recharging time for every worker; it's more important than lunch, it's more important than coffee breaks. Treasure it.

SOCIAL

■ **Do something for someone else each day.**

What better way to take away the pressures of how you react to others, or how others react to you, than to take the initiative and assist them in some way or another?

■ **Mix with winners.**

Spend more time with the people you'd like to be like – positive, stress-free, successful. Do this and you stand a better chance of becoming more like them. (Conversely, avoid negative, depressing people and negative conversation.)

■ **Avoid Type A people.**

It may sound harsh, but if you're a Type A person, stay away from other Type As as much as possible. When you cannot avoid them, at least avoid arguing or competing with them.

■ **Enjoy yourself.**

Above all, look for the positive, humorous, entertaining or even ridiculous sides of what you do.

demand a written job description (which outlines how you will be rewarded and assessed); the layout of your workplace should be altered to allow you access to natural light, and so on.

Yet, the most effective solutions lie with you.

You alone control how you react to work. You alone can guarantee that work is a challenge rather than a trial. The techniques on pages 284–5 are designed just for you.

The Total Effort

My grandmother's sister worked in the laundry of a city hospital for more than forty years. She was still working there well into her eighties. For all those years, she found this hot, repetitive, labour-intensive work to be both stimulating and immensely fulfilling. How could she find it stimulating?

Have you even wondered why your grandmother can crochet away hour after hour, and derive enormous peace and satisfaction from it, yet the same repetitive pastime would drive you around the bend in minutes?

Have you ever wondered why that man at your work can work day in, day out, drilling holes in stainless steel sheets, and never stop whistling and flashing smiles, yet you'd be an irritable wreck after only 10 minutes of that monotony?

Have you ever wondered why the woman down the street can happily take in basket-load after basket-load of other people's ironing, and derive enormous peace and satisfaction from doing so (without having to watch television to distract herself while she irons), yet you go cold at the very thought of pressing more than three blouses at a time?

Is it because they are more limited people than you are? Is it because they have higher 'thresholds of boredom' or lower 'thresholds of expectation' than you? Is it because they're *superior* people to you?

Would you believe that it's none of these reasons? Would you believe that these people simply know, instinctively, a powerful calming technique that you do not?

They do.

The enigma of repetition

At the root of most calming meditation styles you'll find repetition. Indeed, many of the better known meditation techniques employ a device known as a mantra which is, essentially, a word or sound that is repeated over and over and over.

Why is it, then, that this repetition is so calming in meditation yet can be so frustrating and tension-building in other areas?

Workers on assembly lines, for example, are often highly stressed and get little satisfaction from the repetitive nature of their work. People who spend their days ironing garment after garment – often with little appreciation for their efforts – usually find the chore to be the pinnacle of frustration. Data processor operators who key in numbers, day in, day out, are often highly strung and susceptible to stress-related disorders.

What makes one form of repetition calming, while another is its most frustrating opposite?

The answer has nothing to do with the level of job satisfaction or with meditation techniques – it is to do with the amount of control you have, or don't have.

Or *believe* you don't have!

In meditation *you* are calling all the shots: you can stop when you want to, you can go and get a cup of tea when you choose, you can abandon meditation altogether should you so decide. However on the assembly line, at the ironing board or at the data entry keyboard you are denied control; someone else is often in charge, calling the shots, enforcing the repetition.

What follows is a technique designed to take the repetitive or mundane nature of work – let's face it, all work is mundane at some stage or another – and turn it into a calming, fulfilling exercise. Better still, this technique is not limited to work: it is equally as effective for knitting, teaching your children to read, and for long-distance driving or running.

The key to this technique is Total Effort. (Those of you who know anything of Zen will recognise my plagiary.)

Say, for example, you have to hand-paint a high, long brick wall inside a warehouse – 100 metres (330 feet) of plain, tedious brick, with no little arches or windows to amuse you, with no company or conversation to distract you, and no massive bonus waiting at the end to make it all seem worthwhile. If you're in any way like me, you will not be able to imagine a more tedious task. (My apologies to professional painters; I have only admiration for you.)

There are two ways you can approach such a task.

You can do what most people do: remind yourself every 30 seconds what a huge job you have in front of you, how long it is until lunch, how unfortunate you are in having to paint the longest and most boring wall in creation, how you'd rather be outdoors in such perfect weather, and how you're not going to receive a cent for your efforts since you were paid in advance for it June last year. You would not be alone if you chose to look at it that way.

> Dividing your attention creates tension; concentrating your attention on only one thing is not only calming, but is the most efficient way you can function.

But you would be much better off if you chose to look at it another way.

You could start by accepting what is. The task is a given; unless you can change or reject it, it should be made the most of. That being so, the object is to turn it into a calming, creative and fulfilling exercise.

How?

By dedicating yourself to doing the best possible paint job you are humanly capable of. If you did make this commitment, you'd immerse yourself in the detail – as a perfectionist would – so that not a crevice was ignored; you'd ensure the surface preparation was as free from blemish as you could manage; you'd make each brush stroke as even and as thorough as you could manage; you'd be careful not to spill a drop on the concrete floor below. (Naturally, if you were a professional painter, all of the aforementioned would have to be done within the constraints of time and budget.) You would be immersed in the effort.

Wonder of wonders … within only minutes, you'd be more calm and relaxed than you thought you were meant to be at work – even with all the concentration you had been applying. You would find that time flew and the day passed in an instant. And, most of all, you would derive an unusually high level of satisfaction and fulfilment from having completed a task to the best of your abilities.

Do not be misled by this simplicity of this technique. It works! There are millions of calm and contented people throughout the world who religiously apply this philosophy of total dedication to their daily lives.

My grandmother's sister used it to find stimulation in the hospital laundry; your grandmother used it to find peace and relaxation in her knitting; the whistling factory worker uses it to find satisfaction in his monotonous drilling; you can use it too.

Moreover, you can use it in areas totally unrelated to work. You can use it when reading the paper, when eating lunch, when pruning the hedge.

The important thing is that you use it to make yourself feel calm, relaxed and satisfied at whatever time you choose.

THE TOTAL EFFORT TECHNIQUE

- The key to this is to do only one thing at the one time. And to do it as totally as you possibly can.
  Whatever it is you are doing – cleaning, driving, working – commit to it as thoroughly, as conscientiously, and as skilfully as you can.
- Try to exclude all external stimuli, such as radio or conversation.
- Concentrate on every step of your activity. Concentrate on the detail. Endeavour to do it as effectively as you can.
  Be the best driver on the entire highway. Give your bath the best scrubbing it has ever had – or that you're capable of giving.
- Continue this way until you forget what you are doing and feel calm, relaxed and at peace.

The Worry Hour

Time and time again throughout our lives it's been drummed into us never to put off until tomorrow what we can do today. It is one of the core beliefs of achievers and workaholics, and it is the cornerstone of the work ethic. But as meaningful as this homily might be to most aspects of our lives, there is one where it applies only in the opposite: that's in the area of worry.

I'm sure you'll agree that it makes great sense to postpone worries and anxieties wherever possible. It could be argued that it makes sense to postpone them indefinitely.

This implies, of course, that your worries and anxieties are conscious, rational thoughts – which they seldom are. So how can you *consciously* decide to postpone feelings that, invariably, are products of the *sub-conscious* mind? How can you postpone feelings at all?

A technique I've used with great success over the years – in fact, it is the one technique I use more regularly than any other – is called the Worry Hour.

It's a worry postponing technique.

To be effective, it requires a degree of formality – or, at least a degree of habit. All you have to do is set aside a certain amount of time each

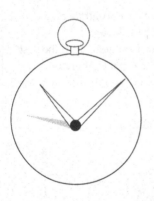

day for worrying. During this time you can be as bitter and as negative as you like, because you will have preconditioned yourself to believe that, at the end of the period, you will be cleansed and relaxed; nine times out of ten, your worries will be gone.

In my case, I not only set aside a certain amount of time, I have also nominated a specific place for it to happen. It's a place I pass every time I go walking – I've designated it the 'stress stretch'. This stretch is not much more than a kilometre in length, and is located in a suburban street of no particular relevance.

Every issue that arises during the day that could turn into a worry I officially postpone to the Worry Hour (or, in my case, the 'stress stretch'). I note my anxieties, I note the parameters of my worries, I record all the details required to make a decision (if a decision is to be made). Then, I do my best to forget about them until my walk that evening. Until the moment I hit the 'stress stretch'.

All along that suburban street flows an outpouring of the worries, anxieties, disappointments, frustrations of the day. It's a miserable few minutes, I can tell you. *But it's only a few minutes.* And, at the end of it – at the end of the 'stress stretch' – my head is clear, my tension gone, my worries removed, and very often my problems are solved.

The beauty of this technique is that you have to do very little except make the initial decision; almost all of the effort is carried out by the subconscious.

Do it regularly and sincerely, and you will be able to dismiss your anxieties at will. There is no faster way to feeling calm than that.

THE WORRY HOUR

- Designate a certain time and place where you can conduct your worry sessions each day. Preferably, this will be away from your work or your home.
- Whenever worries, frustrations, irritations or anxieties arise during the day, postpone them until your worry hour. Consciously take note of them, as well as their details, maybe even writing them in a notebook, with a view to reviewing them in full when the time arrives.
- Devote all of your attention to these concerns for a designated period of time. Do it in the understanding that relief or a solution awaits at the end of the period.
- At the end of the specified worry period, move from that place, and stop thinking about your problems entirely.
- Trust in your subconscious to have the solution you require.

28

TYPE A
TECHNIQUES

Sociologists and medical researchers traditionally like to break the community into convenient categories. In the areas of heart disease and stress management, two of the most spoken-about categorisations are the behavioural/attitudinal types known as 'Type A' and 'Type B'.

These obviously are stereotypes. All people do not fit stereotypes. However, the Type A behaviour patterns described here will not only be familiar to you, but they are also extremely relevant to those who suffer the ill-effects of negative stress.

According to some well-known research programmes, Type A people are significantly more prone to heart disease and stress-induced ailments than Type B. Even though the research studies have been challenged from time to time, you will have to search a long way to find a medical person who will dispute this assertion.

So what is it about Type A people that makes them more prone to stress-related ailments? Why are Type A people so self-destructive? Why have I assumed that the majority of readers of this book are Type A people – and have thus included a section solely on that topic?

The answers to all of those questions are illustrated opposite.

You will find that you, and most people you know, will lean very heavily to one side of the chart or the other.

If most of your characteristics are on the right-hand side, you are a Type B person and can skip the rest of this chapter. You will probably live longer, have a lower disease record, and will suffer less from stress-related problems than your friends on the other side. You may also be a better manager, more efficient at what you do, and more able to cope with the ups and downs of everyday life.

The rest of us, unfortunately, have a long way to go.

Most of the techniques in this book will work equally as well for

TYPE A PERSONALITIES

- Create their own stress
- Are achievement oriented
- Are highly competitive
- Are usually assertive
- Set themselves difficult targets
- Set themselves difficult deadlines
- Attempt several things at once
- Push themselves to the limits
- Are always in a hurry
- Are Impatient
- Are easily bored
- Use clipped, aggressive speech
- Breathe faster and shallower
- Display 'tense' body language
- Are self-centred
- Forget details, make mistakes
- Consume too much coffee, etc.
- Feel guilty about relaxing

TYPE B PERSONALITIES

- Have stress created for them
- Are interested in 'living', not 'having'
- If ambitious, are not over-competitive
- Are more easy-going than Type A
- Are realistic about what is achievable
- Set reasonable deadlines
- Approach tasks methodically
- Know their limits
- Are relaxed
- Are less driven, less obsessive
- Can find interest in most things
- Speak slower, communicate better
- Breathe slower and deeper
- Display 'relaxed' body language
- Are more outgoing
- Are organised, make fewer mistakes
- Consume modestly
- Relish the opportunity to unwind

Type A or Type B people. Following, however, are some that have been specifically designed to counter the pressures that Type A people are so determined to heap upon themselves.

In 1989, an experiment was conducted using these techniques on a group of very stressed and very cynical executives from large corporations. In most cases, the results were not only extremely positive, but directly attributable to the techniques employed.

You will find these techniques do not expect you to change from the type of person you are – though this may be a positive step. You will also pleased to note that they've been specially designed to conform to the more common Type A expectations.

But best of all, they work.

Pretend to be Type B

Although there's no need to cover this in detail again, a powerful technique for emulating Type B behaviour characteristics is the Let's Pretend Technique covered on page 112.

In this instance, however, instead of conjuring up an image of yourself as simply calm, relaxed and stress-free, you can conjure up an image of yourself as a Type B personality.

Once that image is set in your mind, it simply becomes a matter of pretending to be a Type B person, and pretending that those who come in contact with you recognise you as such a person.

Give Yourself Permission

Type A people like to think of themselves as being in control. As you would imagine, exercising control requires a considerable effort from the *conscious* mind.

Imagine what would happen, then, if you made a conscious decision to grant yourself permission to relax.

You would still see yourself as being in charge. But you would not be bossing your subconscious around, ordering it to relax (which you know is a sure way of achieving nothing because the subconscious will not be ordered, it must be charmed). By using the following technique, your subconscious will respond just the way you want it to.

The technique is very simple. It requires you to study the comparison chart on page 293 a little closer.

When you rise in the morning, find a quiet place by yourself for a few minutes and say out loud: 'For 5 minutes in every hour, I give myself permission to relax and be more like a Type B person.'

Think about what this means. *Repeat it at least ten times.*

(It is Type A behaviour to protest that you can't afford 5 minutes in every hour. By taking this 5 minutes, you will be substantially more effective in the remainder of that hour.)

Now, throughout your day, find somewhere quiet – when you're driving, in the bathroom, on your way to lunch – and repeat those words another ten times.

Do this at least five times throughout the day.

Essentially, that's all you have to do. Your subconscious will do the rest.

If, after a couple of days, you feel you are not becoming sufficiently relaxed by using this technique, use it *in conjunction with* one of the techniques that follow.

GIVE YOURSELF PERMISSION

- Study the difference between Type A and Type B behaviour (page 293).
- First thing in the morning, find a quiet place and say the following to yourself out loud: 'For 5 minutes in every hour, I give myself permission to relax and to be more like a Type B person.'
- Think about what this means. Repeat it 10 times.
- At least **5 times** throughout the day, find a quiet place and repeat this entire exercise.
- Your subconscious will do the rest.
  [Note If, after a couple of days, you feel you are not becoming sufficiently relaxed by using this technique, use it in conjunction with one of the others that follow.]

An Hour of Type B

Type A people want to do everything better, faster and more successfully than everyone else. This is usually what drives them.

Yet studies show that Type B people – even though they may lack some of the drive and ambition of their Type A counterparts – are usually better leaders, better managers, better communicators, and more efficient at most things they do. All other things being equal, of course.

It makes good Type A sense, therefore, to be Type B. If your subconscious works like mine, it has already seen the appeal in this exquisite logic.

Let's start by assuming that it's too radical a change for you to become a Type B type altogether. In any event, being a Type A personality you would probably approach this task in an obsessive, totally Type A manner, thus negating all of the potential benefits.

Instead, let's choose a certain part of every day, or every week, or every month, where you can masquerade as a Type B person. Say, for example, you decide that every day between 9 and 10 a.m., you're going to display Type B characteristics (which you've re-read on page 293).

It is important to utilise these characteristics intuitively, not consciously.

To do this, you will first need to imagine what it's like to be a Type B person – how it looks, sounds, acts and feels. You can do this by conjuring up an image of yourself displaying these characteristics on your 'big screen'.

Somewhere in that image is one distinct, physical element that you can appropriate at any time. Maybe it's an undone collar button (versus the stiff buttoned-up look you adopt each day); maybe it's a brightly coloured neck scarf (versus the formal-looking pearls you wear every day); maybe it's simply a complete absence of a wristwatch. Let's assume you choose the last. *Physically* remove your wristwatch.

Now, take another look at your image on the 'big screen'. Notice how much more Type B you feel without that wristwatch. Notice how deadlines seem not to loom so threateningly, how you have plenty of time to complete your work, how you do one thing at a time *and enjoy it.* Notice how relaxed and calm you feel.

When you feel you are experiencing that Type B experience to the maximum, 'turn up' the image and sound on your big screen.

Now, every day when it's time to become a Type B person, all you have to do is remove your wristwatch, recall the Type B characteristics, and leave the rest to your subconscious.

AN HOUR OF TYPE B

- Mark off in your diary the time when you're going to emulate a Type B personality. Start with one specific hour in each day.
- Read closely the difference between Type A and Type B behaviour.
- Remember the Conditions of Calm.
- On your 'big screen' conjure up an image of yourself if you were a Type B person. Note the way you're standing, the type of clothes you're wearing – in each instance, this will be different to what you are doing and wearing now.
- Choose one of these physical elements that you can appropriate. Say, for example, your Type B image does not wear a watch.
- Physically remove your watch.
- Now take a closer look at your image on the screen. Notice how deadlines no longer seem so threatening. How you have plenty of time to complete your work. How you do one thing at a time and *enjoy* it. How relaxed you feel.
- Now 'turn up' the picture and the sound. Stay with that relaxed feeling for a couple of minutes.
- Every day, spend at least one hour being a Type B personality. All you have to do is remove your watch, recall those positive Type B characteristics, and your subconscious will take care of the rest.

'No' Can Be Positive

Type A people are their own worst enemies. When it comes to work-loads, life goals, favours, domestic chores, they invariably end up taking on more than they can sensibly handle.

Why? Do they want to be able to say they are overworked? Are they the world's worst planners? Do they seriously overestimate their capacities? Are they so inefficient that they will always be unable to complete the tasks they set for themselves?

Often, the answer to all of the above is a resounding 'yes'.

I believe, however, that above all else, Type A people share one major failing: they can't say 'no'. They can't say no to extra workloads. They can't say no to requests for favours or assistance. They can't say no to invitations.

Yet anyone who faces time problems will agree that the greatest time wasters (that is, the greatest stressors) are not the major projects, but the minor ones, the ones you probably shouldn't be doing in the first place.

It is no secret that, in business, most damage comes from lots of small problems as opposed to one large one. Nor is it a secret that most breakdowns are the product of lots of minor issues rather than one major one.

It follows, therefore, that if you could avoid these minor issues, that you would be much better equipped to do a good job on the major ones.

But how? How do you say 'no'? When do you say 'no'?

While I would dearly love to formularise this for you, there are no simple answers to this issue other than the following.

a Set goals, targets and outcomes.
b Only take on what will help you achieve those goals, targets and outcomes. (That is, say 'no' to everything else.)
c Ignore all Type A arguments to the contrary.

Set goals, targets and outcomes

This is the most difficult task most Type A personalities face in life. I suspect many Type A people are that way, simply because they cannot establish specific goals, targets and outcomes for themselves.

But you can.

Even if those you set are less than perfect, or are downright flawed, they will be better than having none at all. Besides, you can always revise.

The starting point is your outcome: at the end of the process, what will you have achieved? What will you be? How will you feel?

Outcomes are not goals. Outcomes are not desires. Outcomes are goals and desires that are realised. Outcomes are always spoken about in the present ('I am so wealthy and successful that I will never have to work, and will never have to fill out a cheque butt again'). Outcomes are always expressed in positive terms ('I am relaxed and happy' – *not* 'I am free from stress'). Outcomes are best determined by examining pictures on your 'big screen'.

Goals and targets, on the other hand, are simply steps to achieve along the way.

Take out your notebook again and, at the top of the page, write your outcome (for life, work, relationship, or whatever you choose). Beneath that write your goals and targets. Quantify them as best you can.

Keep this page in a safe place. Refer to it often.

Take on only what helps you achieve those goals, targets and outcomes

Now, whenever someone asks you to do something you hadn't planned for, you have three clear choices.

a Say 'yes' if it will help you achieve your outcome and if it can be accommodated within your goals and targets.
b Say 'yes' if it will help someone in a serious matter and it doesn't impact negatively on your outcome or goals.
c Say 'no'.

At the end of the day, though, the more things you can say 'no' to, the better off you'll be.

Resist all Type A arguments to the contrary

The arguments go like this.

■ If I say 'no' I will be perceived as being negative.
  ANSWER: *Say, 'Sorry, I have too much to do. I cannot find the time'.*

■ If I say 'no' I will be hindering my advancement/business/relationship prospects.

ANSWER: *Those prospects will already be defined in your outcomes and goals. If advancement is your goal, therefore, you will obviously say 'yes'.*

■ I can never think of a single suitable outcome, there are so many things I want to achieve.

ANSWER: *Write an outcome for every aspect of your life – work, relationships, health, you name it.*

■ It's no use writing down my outcome or goals, I'll almost certainly change my mind.

ANSWER: *When you change your mind, rewrite your outcome and goals. You're the only one keeping points, you know.*

'NO' CAN BE POSITIVE

■ Set goals, targets and outcomes.
'Outcomes' are goals and desires that are realised.
Outcomes are always spoken about in the present ('I am so wealthy and successful that I will never have to work again'), are expressed in positive terms, and are best determined by examining pictures on your 'big screen'.
Goals and targets are simply steps to achieve along the way.

■ Write your outcome at the top of a page, set your goals and targets beneath it.

■ Evaluate all requests and new activities in light of what you've written on your page. Only take on what will help you achieve those goals, targets and outcomes. Say 'no' to everything else.

■ Resist all Type A arguments to the contrary.

Child's Play

Children have a natural ability that few adults (particularly Type A adults) can equal. Instinctively, children know how to be spontaneous, how to laugh and have a good time, how to accept life as it is. And, on top of that, they're not afraid to make mistakes.

Is it any wonder that children generally do not suffer the stresses and anxieties that adults do?

If you can become more like a child – especially at those times where you are at your Type A worst – you will be able to access those childlike attributes that counter the effects of stress.

> If you can become more like a child – especially at those times where you are at your Type A worst – you will be able to access those childlike attributes that counter the effects of stress.

If you can think of yourself as a child and an adult at the same time, you will enjoy the simple events of your life without being bored or intimidated by them. You will be able to approach your problems in a less serious way, and to make fun of all your heavy responsibilities – without neglecting them, of course.

You can achieve this by combining three different approaches: physical, attitudinal and behavioural.

The **physical** approach is the easiest; it also has a major influence over your attitude. All it requires is for you to carry about a physical, though not necessarily visible, accoutrement of child's play – preferably something that relates to your past. Perhaps you wear a pair of Donald Duck socks or underpants. Maybe you carry a water pistol (a toy-looking one, please) in your briefcase, or a bag of marbles. What is important is that this toy, or garment, or whatever you choose, has no practical, high-tech or brain-hurting purpose; it is there for the game, for the novelty, to remind you of what you used to be like.

Type A people will have a tendency to ignore this physical aspect of the technique, preferring instead to concentrate on the problem-solving nature of the 'attitudinal approach'. Try not to react like a Type A person in this instance, and you will be well rewarded.

Armed with this physical reminder of a more carefree time of your life, you can now concentrate on the **attitudinal** side. To do this, all you have to do is view everything that threatens you through a child's eyes.

If you're worried about an avalanche of deadlines, imagine how you would look at them if you were a small child. Even though you may still approach them in a professional, workmanlike way, you would not feel overwhelmed by them.

If you're worried about what others might think of you, or something you've done, consider those events through a child's eyes. They don't look so serious now, do they?

Researchers now believe that laughter is one of the cheapest and most powerful therapies at every person's disposal. The act of laughing helps to stabilise your blood pressure and to improve circulation. In some ways it's like aerobics on the inside.

Finally, the **behavioural** approach; once again, this will have an impact on your attitude.

All you have to do is give into some 'childish' impulse, or perform some 'childish' act, at least once an hour. (This is much easier than it sounds for most Type A people. You have to work at it.)

Perhaps it's simply pulling a series of silly faces. Maybe you'll want to stand on your desk for 30 seconds. Or act out a small scene where you call your boss 'Big Ears'.

No one has to witness this and it shouldn't serve any practical purpose other than to remind you of a more carefree time of life. *And if it causes you to laugh, or to expend physical energy, so much the better.*

CHILD'S PLAY

- Carry about a physical reminder of a more carefree time of your life. It may be a toy, or a garment, or a game – ensure that it has no practical purpose or intention. (If you didn't have a pleasant childhood, carry something that reminds you of the childhood you would like to have had.)
- With this physical reminder close by, concentrate on seeing your day-to-day life through a child's eyes. Look for the light-hearted side of 'disasters' (most children would not take them seriously for a second). Look for the fun side of problem-solving or deadline-meeting.
- Do something 'childish' and ridiculous at least once an hour. No one has to see you and it doesn't have to serve any practical purpose. And if it causes you to laugh, or to expend physical energy, so much the better.

Call It a Day

One of the crosses that Type A people have to bear is that they alone are responsible for earning the living, running the business, managing the home, raising the children, choosing the Christmas presents, planning the menu.

Or so they believe.

One of the more effective means of dealing with this Type A belief system is to contain the various tasks of the day.

Your occupation, for example, usually represents a field day for Type A abuses. Not only can you

> Type B people go home at night and think of things other than work. They go out and enjoy themselves. They indulge in 'time wasting' recreational pursuits. They throw themselves into family activities and work on their relationships. Next day, they return to work and pick up the threads from the previous day.

worry and be obsessed all day long, but you can take your worries home, think about them all night, and be even more worried.

Type B people, on the other hand, go home at night and think of other things. They go out and enjoy themselves. They indulge in 'time wasting' recreational pursuits. They throw themselves into family activities and work on their relationships. Next day, they return to work and pick up the threads from the previous day.

Surprise, surprise: this Type B behaviour works. Not only are the people who use it more relaxed about their work, they are usually more efficient as well (probably as a result of being more relaxed.)

How can you contain your Type A compulsions so that you, too, can switch off after a day's work? So that you, too, will know when to call it a day?

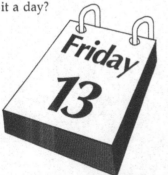

Simple. Most people travel to and from work in the same way, day in, day out. As you're travelling to work, you can indulge your Type A needs to the fullest: think about work, make notes, worry about the day ahead.

But when you're travelling *home from work*, reserve your thoughts for something else. Make a rule that says

CALL IT A DAY

- On leaving your workplace, say to yourself: 'I give myself the night off, to relax and indulge myself'. Or: 'I give myself the night off, to relax and enjoy my relationship'. Say this 10 times. Aloud if possible.
- All the way home, plan how you're going to make the most of indulging yourself, or enjoying your relationship. Plan it in detail. Think about the positive steps you are going to take to achieve it. Think about how good and how relaxed you're going to feel after you have done it.
- Make the most of your night off, knowing that you will be more relaxed and better at your work tomorrow.

you stay at work until you complete what you can complete for the day, then work is over.

You are free.

The moment you walk out of the door of your work, say to yourself, 'I give myself the night off, to relax and indulge myself.' Yes, it is permissible, even advisable, for a hard-working Type A person to indulge him or herself.

Alternately, you could say, 'I give myself the night off, to relax and enjoy my relationship'.

Repeat this ten times. Aloud, if you can get away with it.

Now start planning how you're going to make the most of indulging yourself, or enjoying your relationship. Plan it in detail. Think about the positive steps you are going to take to achieve it. Think about how good and how relaxed you're going to feel after you have done it. (You'll also feel much better for it at work tomorrow, but try not to think about that.)

By the time you've planned all this, you should be home.

Then, go ahead, indulge yourself.

This concept of knowing when to call it a day is also beneficial in other areas of Type A activities such as knowing when to give up on a project, knowing when to quit from an unsatisfying job or relationship, knowing when to stop taking on new activities.

Alone Time

Alone time. Without it, you will worry more, you will be more prone to stress-related problems, your health will be impaired, and your life will probably be shortened – reasons enough to give it some serious consideration right now.

Sometimes it is a great use of time to do absolutely nothing. While many Type A people may be loners, few permit themselves any quality 'alone time', where they sit by themselves and do absolutely nothing.

Alone Time is simply a period of time you set aside *each day* for being. For seeking release from the pressures of everyday life. For enjoying your own self.

Generally, this Alone Time will take 20–30 minutes. It can be first thing in the morning, last thing at night, or any time in between. During your Alone Time, no company is permitted, no stimuli are permitted, no thinking about work or other problems is permitted.

Whether you use this time to apply any of the techniques in this book, to meditate, to practise Power Breathing, or to sit and stare at the wall is unimportant at this stage. What is important is that you make the commitment to spending the time, doing nothing, each day.

Equally as important is to schedule some Alone Time during your day. Allow a 15-minute buffer zone between engagements, to give yourself a little stress-free space.

To the Type A way of thinking,

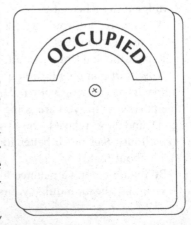

this concept will be the zenith of time wasting. When the Type A person has an hour free, or 15 minutes free, that time will be spent 'usefully' – watching the news, catching up with correspondence.

But consider this: *without* Alone Time, you will worry more, you will be more prone to stress-related problems, your health will be impaired, and your life will probably be shortened. Aren't these reasons enough to give it serious consideration right now?

ALONE TIME

- Choose at least one 20–30 minute period, once a day, that you designate 'Alone Time'. Permit no company, no stimuli, no thinking about work or other problems.
- Use this time to apply any of the techniques in this book, to meditate, to practise Power Breathing, or to sit and stare at the wall. Do it regularly and you will worry less, you will be less prone to stress-related problems, your health will be improved, and your life will probably be lengthened.

Talk To Yourself

The internal dialogue (the mental words you use when you're thinking things through) that most Type A people use is peppered with expressions like 'must', 'have to', 'ought to', 'got to' and so on.

When you listen to such people speak, even their external dialogue sounds the same. 'I *have* to finish this by nine:' 'I *must* go to the dentist.' 'I *should* trim the ivy from the front of the house.' 'I *have* to be more circumspect in my conversation with strangers.'

Note the instructions they give themselves. These are known as pressure instructions: constant reminders that you must do and achieve more and more. They create pressure. They create stress. Not only do they set an endless agenda, but they perpetuate the feeling that there's always more to be done. You will never have to reflect and be satisfied with what you've achieved, because there is always something else hanging over your head.

Type A people thrive on pressure instructions; using them feeds their tension and anxiety.

Yet, simply by choosing different words for your internal (and external) dialogue, you can eliminate all of the pressures associated with this type of language.

How do you do it? Substitute 'choose to' for 'have to' and you will feel an immediate change in your attitude. Tell yourself: 'I *choose* to finish this by nine' . . . 'I *choose* to go to the dentist' . . . 'I *choose* to trim the ivy from the front of the house' . . . and you will be a changed person.

Perhaps you're the type who would profit more from being let off the 'have to' hook altogether. If this is the case, substitute 'can' for 'have to'. Now, you would tell yourself: 'I *can* finish this by nine' . . . ' 'I *can* go to the dentist' . . . 'I *can* trim the ivy from the front of the house'.

Either way, this new freedom will allow you to feel much more relaxed and comfortable about your duties and your day.

TALK TO YOURSELF

- To remove the Type A pressures in your internal and external dialogue, substitute 'choose to' for 'have to'.
  'I *choose* to finish this by nine' – as opposed to 'I have to finish this by nine'. 'I *choose* to go to the dentist' – as opposed to 'I have to go to the dentist'.
- If you want to be under even less pressure, substitute 'can' instead of 'have to'.
- Use this language, not only for internal dialogue, but for your conversation as well.

Take the Long Road Home

One of the easiest, yet most profound, ways of achieving deep relaxation is to allow yourself to take it easy when you least want to do it.

While 'taking it easy' is meaningless when you are wasting time, it comes into its fore when you are most driven and under pressure.

Next time the weight of the world is on your shoulders, try this: instead of rushing home from work after your gruelling 14-hour day, drive home via a different, longer route. Give yourself permission to take your time, to check out the scenery, to listen to the radio.

Alternatively, leave the car at work and try taking a bus. Spend your time absorbing the differences of that world, the variations that life has to offer. You counter the effects of stress by broadening the perspective of your life, by taking the time to see and experience the bigger picture. By expanding your experiences, you expand your world. And by expanding your world, your little anxieties seem less important.

Even if it's only for half an hour on the way home from work, this is a cheap and simple way of getting off the treadmill, which is a sure and simple way of escaping the stresses of everyday life.

29

THE CALM TECHNIQUE

Such is the power of the technique that follows that I have written an entire book on the topic. Not surprisingly, it is called *the Calm Technique*. Part of what this book is about is a sure technique for finding peace and harmony in a troubled world.

The Calm Technique is a simple exercise that anyone can master and apply.

With a minimum of effort, you will discover a way that will allow you to be more positive, more creative, more alive, more tolerant, more able to cope . . . and, of course, more calm.

Use it regularly, and it will change your life. Nothing is surer.

The Calm Technique is, for want of a better word, meditation. Yet it requires no particular spiritual belief or understanding, and nor does it subscribe to any particular philosophy or way of life. As the title of the original book said, it is 'meditation without magic or mysticism'.

So, what is meditation?

There are a hundred definitions, most of which I find either precious or obtuse.

Quite simply, it is the process of stilling the mind – suspending the process of conscious thought – so that you can simply 'be'. As Buddha is reputed to have instructed, 'Don't meditate; be in meditation.'

During meditation you exist purely in the moment: nothing can distract you, no worries about the past or concerns for the future; your mind and your emotions are at rest. Many believe this is the most perfect state possible for one's consciousness or awareness.

The effect on your physiology

Meditation is not an experience, as such. It is simply 'being', perhaps not even aware of that state. However, despite its subtlety, it brings about a series of distinct and unique physiological processes.

While you are in the meditative state, there is a dramatic change in the pattern of your brainwaves. There is an increase in the slow alpha waves – which are usually only present when you are wide awake and relaxed. Yet, at the same time as these alpha waves are present, there is a definite presence of delta waves which usually occur only in the deepest sleep. *So your brainwaves indicate a state of mind that is highly alert at the same time that it is in deep relaxation.* To compound the paradox, there is virtually no rapid eye movement (REM) – an indication of sleep and dreaming – during the meditative state.

More pertinent to this book, perhaps, is the effect it has on your metabolism. Your oxygen consumption decreases even further than it does in deep sleep. Your heartbeat and blood pressure decrease almost as dramatically. The lactate level (which increases during stress) in your bloodstream decreases by up to 50 per cent, nearly four times faster than in a state of deep relaxation.

These unique physiological states are the *opposite* to those you experience during moments of stress or anxiety.

And this is why meditation produces such a profound sense of peace, harmony and wellbeing.

How do you do it?

Despite the fact that many organisations have devoted their existence to teaching it, and despite the fact that I have written books and conducted countless seminars talking about it, meditation is exquisitely simple.

It is not altogether different to any other trancelike state you might be familiar with: running a long-distance race, taking a long bus ride, knitting a scarf, listening to the waves.

To achieve this state at will is a simple matter of focusing – focusing the mind on one thing so that it excludes all others.

Some meditation techniques would have you focus on a physical object, or on a complex series of actions (as in tai chi). For purposes of simplicity, the Calm Technique requires you to concentrate on a sound.

The sound can be anything you choose. I suggest that it is the sound of your own voice speaking a single word – any word – over and over again.

Once again, for the purposes of this exercise, let's say the word is 'Calm'.

Most meditation techniques claim superiority over others because of the specific sense they use to focus the attention – a sound, a fixed object (internal or external), breathing, a feeling, an intellectual concept, physical exercises. This is hogwash. Each individual habitually favours one 'modality' over another – visual, auditory, kinaesthetic, intellectual – which means that a meditation technique favouring that particular modality will *seem* more profound to them. However each of us has the capacity to use all modalities. So each of the meditation styles are, theoretically, as effective as one another.

That's all you have to do. That is the total process. One word repeated (in your mind) over and over again for a period of 20 or 30 minutes. And when your attention strays – which it will – you simply guide it back to that repeated word or sound as you become aware of the fact.

Even as briefly as I have described it, the Calm Technique will work for you as long as you remember four things:

a   it is meant to be as easy as it appears
b   the experience in itself does not have to be anything special
c   it is not a test of concentration or will power
d   those who approach with an open mind will almost always find a solution to their problems during meditation.

For a more complete understanding, read the book, *the Calm Technique*.

THE CALM TECHNIQUE

- Remember the Conditions of Calm. Low lights, comfortable clothes, comfortable temperature.
- Perform Power Breathing for a minute or so. Close your eyes, listen to your breath.
- Quietly say the word 'Calm' to yourself. Listen to yourself speak. Choose whatever rhythm you feel comfortable with as you repeat it over and over.
- Now 'hear' yourself saying it, without uttering a sound. 'Hear' the word coming from inside your head, directly back from where your eyes are.
- Continue 'hearing' this word, over and over again, for at least 20 minutes. When you discover yourself wandering, gently go back to 'reciting' that word. Don't force yourself; don't worry if you can't do it well – it does not matter.
- After 20 minutes or so, gradually bring your attention back to the present. Sit and wait a few minutes, as you become more alert and awake.
- For a more complete understanding, read the book *the Calm Technique.*

CRISIS

30

CRISIS –
WHAT TO DO

In researching this book, I have become only too aware of the minor nature of most people's stressors; problems that seem insurmountable today often fade into obscurity tomorrow, or when you meet someone whose problems are unmistakably worse.

> The effects of long-term negative stress brought about by 'minor' issues can be just as damaging as those brought about by major issues.

Such an understanding, of course, does not lessen the pain or impact of our troubles. Indeed, the health and emotional repercussions of 'minor' problems, or even undefined problems and anxieties, can be equally as toxic as those we recognise as 'major'. In other words, the effects of long-term negative stress brought about by 'minor' issues can be just as damaging as those brought about by major issues.

While this book has demonstrated many ways of finding immediate relief from the effects of everyday stress, major crises may require a different approach.

What is a major crisis?

Grief, serious illness, physical or emotional trauma, extreme career or relationship issues, arrest – I have no doubt you will recognise them when they strike. In such an unfortunate eventuality, you may find you need additional remedies to those we have addressed throughout this book.

To begin with, though, adopt the 'Calm in Crisis' measures.

CALM IN CRISIS

1 Remove your shoes.
2 Stay warm.
3 Don't even *think* about cigarettes, coffee or alcohol.
4 Begin Power Breathing.
5 Listen to each breath, concentrate on your breathing; do it as perfectly as you can manage.
6 Seek help.

Help

The National Trauma Clinic says that one of the biggest mistakes people make when trying to deal with a crisis is to try to handle it alone.

Seeking help is not a sign of weakness. Seek it from a friend, a spiritual advisor, or from one of the many crisis counsellors you will find in the phone book (most tend not to charge for their services).

There are enormous, sometimes even life-saving, benefits to be derived from an intimate discussion with another. Whether that discussion draws useful advice or not is seldom the issue; the real benefit comes from sharing your experience and in receiving encouragement to continue.

If you are at a loss as to whom you can turn, look under 'Crisis' in the telephone directory. The directories of most cities have a listing under that heading.

INDEX